SLEEP APNEA

Health Benefits That You Get From a Good Night's Sleep

(It Will Take You Into a Pain Free Sleep Study)

Julie Dupre

Published by Tomas Edwards

Sleep Apnea: Health Benefits That You Get From a Good Night's Sleep (It Will Take You Into a Pain Free Sleep Study)

ISBN 978-1-990268-38-0

Legal & Disclaimer

The information contained in this book is not designed to replace or take the place of any form of medicine or professional medical advice. The information in this book has been provided for educational and entertainment purposes only.

The information contained in this book has been compiled from sources deemed reliable, and it is accurate to the best of the Author's knowledge; however, the Author cannot guarantee its accuracy and validity and cannot be held liable for any errors or omissions. Changes are periodically made to this book. You must consult your doctor or get professional medical advice before using any of the suggested remedies, techniques, or information in this book.

Upon using the information contained in this book, you agree to hold harmless the Author from and against any damages, costs, and expenses, including any legal fees potentially resulting from the application of any of the information provided by this guide. This disclaimer applies to any damages or injury caused by the use and application, whether directly or indirectly, of any advice or information presented, whether for breach of contract, tort, negligence, personal injury, criminal intent, or under any other cause of action.

You agree to accept all risks of using the information presented inside this book. You need to consult a professional medical practitioner in order to ensure you are both able and healthy enough to participate in this program.

Table of Contents

Introduction

This book contains proven steps and strategies on how to identify, observe, diagnose, and treat Sleep Apnea. This book has further listed the different types of Sleep Apnea, how do they manifest and what are its symptoms. Not only this, but you will also find some useful information about some new therapies and treatments associated with Sleep Apnea. All these treatments and methods require expert medical advice and observation.

Sleep Apnea is becoming common these days. As more and more people are turning obese, the risks associated with it are also increasing. And Sleep Apnea is also an after effect of obesity. You will gain a lot of clarity after going through this book on Sleep Apnea. Most of the time, we are unaware of the basic symptoms of any disease, and it is here that I have talked about every known reported symptom of Sleep Apnea. As it is said that early diagnosis is the key to getting guaranteed treatment.

So, make sure that you read this book on Sleep Apnea and understand what it is and how best to tackle Sleep Apnea.

Thanks again for downloading this book, I hope you enjoy it!

Chapter 1: How To Sleep Better With Peaceful Of Mind

Most people who are reading this book are going to want to know about the actions that they can take in order to find a deeper and more satisfying sleep at night. There are many simple things that a person can do in order to get a good night's sleep and here are a few of them. Many sleep disorders that we have already discussed may need the help of a physician in order to make sure that your health is maintained. A chronic fatigue is a symptom of a more significant physical issue and needs to be addressed but if you are simply not sleeping as soundly and consistently as you would like there are some simple do's and don'ts that will help you recapture the night.

One of the first things that a person needs to do is to start to keep track of the sleeping patterns that they are experiencing each day. This is easily accomplished by starting a sleep journal. This will be a record that can help a person identify their sleep patterns and the sleeping disorders that they might be suffering from and how to fight it. Keep this handy notebook right next to your bed and keep it diligently each day.

The first data that should be collected for the journal is going to be the times that you go to bed and the time that you wake up each day. Do not record the times before hand, write it down in the morning after you have gotten up for the day. Then make a note of the total hours of sleep that you experienced that night, 8 hours, 6 hours etc. Underneath each basic entry then it is a place for a recap of the sleeping experience. If you had trouble sleeping describe what you did or were thinking about before your fell asleep. Examples would be, closed eyes and thought about work or had a glass of milk, listened to a recorded book.

One of the most important aspects of the sleep journal is to make sure to note all of the food that you had eaten prior to going to bed and the time that you consumed it. This is not a diet journal so there is no need to deceive yourself. Keeping an accurate record of the foods eaten and the times may hold a vital piece of evidence that will help solve your sleeping problem. Along with the food, it is important to record what your feelings and moods were are you headed to bed that night. These can be just as illuminate as the foods that you eat when it comes time to find the cause of your sleeping problem. Finally there should be a strict record kept about any drugs or alcohol that was consumed and the timing of that use.

All of this information will allow you to combine and create a picture of the sleeping patterns that exist in your life and all of the factors that might be affecting you. The sleep journal will allow you to analyze your behavior more objectively and to see if patterns are emerging as you struggle for sleep each night. If eating at a certain time makes your stay awake or if the feelings that you are experience before sleep have a negative or positive effect on you. Making changes can come once you recognize the problems that exist. Identifying your problems and being honest about them is the first step to finding peaceful, restful and rejuvenating sleep each night.

Once all of your information has been gathered then it is time to look at what else can be done in order to help ourselves sleep on a consistent basis and there are many simple things to do in order to achieve this. As human beings we are by nature creatures of habit. It is important to establish consistent sleep routines so that our bodies and our minds become used to this daily rebooting of our systems. Go to sleep and get up at the same time each and every day even on the weekends. If you are varying the time you go to sleep each day, it isn't a wonder that your body doesn't know when it is time to perform or shut down.

The next suggestion is common sense but many people simply ignore it because they feel like they have to. Allow time each day to get the sleep that your require to be rested and perform at your best each day. This can be a major life change for some people. It is important to realize that you deserve to be treated well. Whatever you are doing it is not more important than your health because once your health is gone then so are you. All of the work that seemed so important won't seem so important at the end of your life. Sleep needs to be a priority for your health.

As we discussed before, make sure that it is dark, cool and comfortable where you sleep. This will eliminate distractions and lead you to finding a comfortable and sound night's sleep. This can be a simple lifestyle change, if you realize from your journal that the it is too hot in your room then lower the temperature. You can also move your bed from one area of the room to another, which might provide better lighting or noise protection. These are simple life changes that can bring sound sleep back into your life today.

Shut down the power. There is a common belief that having smart phones, computer tablets or even watching television in bed can harm your sleeping patterns. Many experts advise removing the television from the bedroom because it adds nothing to your sleeping patterns. The associations that we make with a location can cause us to perform to those expectations. If you watch television in bed then your mind might associate bed with entertainment and not bring sound sleep to you.

The smart phone is a creature that is new to sleep problems. Tuning it off at night is a challenge for many people simply can't handle. On the physical level it is believed that the lights from the screen or even the electrical pulse the phone produces can be unhealthy for people and definitely detrimental to great sleeping habits. On the mental level our minds have become so attached to the gaining of information the turning the phone off at night creates anxiety that can take away from sleep. In effect, people are so worried about missing a staus update or a Tweet that they leave their phone on all night long. The fear of cutting this tether of information can cause an anxiety and sleeping disorder all of its own. This type of lifestyle change can be hard but being able to cut the cord of technology to sleep is a great idea. If someone needs to get in touch with you it will wait until morning.

One of the things that you should not do is to treat your insomnia with sleeping pills. For a short time, under a doctor's care the use of drugs for sleeping problems could be acceptable but for the long term a person shouldn't take a sleeping pill to get a good night's sleep. When you take drugs to provide sleep a person is most often addressing the symptom of the problem and not the problem itself. As we discussed before, an inability to sleep is often a symptom of anxiety, depression or a physical ailment that needs to be addressed. In the short term for one night, a sleeping pill might be ok but make sure that they are never taken with alcohol, because this combination can be deadly.

It is important to make sure that our sleep is valued as much as our physical activity or any other aspect of our life. Take the time to learn how to get a good night's sleep and you will be rewarded with a higher quality of life.

Chapter 2: Insomnia And Medical Causes

The sleep disturbances noted in chapter 1 can and do cause bouts of insomnia but there are other causes. It is important to know if your insomnia is caused by an underlying medical condition. Many medical conditions note insomnia as a symptom and some medication can also cause bouts of insomnia.

The steps in this book can help alleviate insomnia brought on by a medical condition or medication only if the medical condition is treated and the medication changed or stopped. It is important to check with your doctor if you suffer from bouts of insomnia or long term insomnia.

Knowing the causes for your sleeplessness can go a long way to returning you to a regular, healthy sleep cycle.

Non-24 sleep–wake disorder is a chronic sleep disturbance suffered by those who are blind or living in an area with an irregular light/dark cycle in nature. The odd light/dark cycle or the inability to see the light/dark cycle can result in a circadian rhythm problem. This causes the person to wake or sleep at the wrong times during the day.

Non-24-hour sleep-wake disorder should be diagnosed because it can result in long term insomnia if left untreated. Treating this condition usually returns the circadian rhythm to normal and if it was treated early enough, insomnia will improve on its own.

Non-24 is just one example of a condition that triggers insomnia; others include:

Chronic pain

Asthma

Hyperthyroidism

Nasal and sinus allergies

Arthritis

Gastrointestinal issues

Parkinson's disease

Chronic pain makes it difficult for the sufferer to fall asleep and stay asleep. When chronic pain occurs during sleep it will cause the sufferer to wake up; this constant arousal from sleep can cause bouts of insomnia. Reliving the pain for the entire night will go a long way to resolving the secondary insomnia.

14

Asthma left undiagnosed or untreated can disrupt sleep. When sleep is disrupted several times a night due to asthma, it becomes difficult to fall asleep and stay asleep.

Alleviating the asthma can help resolve the insomnia. Another problem for asthma sufferers is the inhaler. Many inhalers contain stimulants, these stimulants can cause insomnia and disrupt healthy, restful sleep.

Hyperthyroidism is a condition that causes the sufferers system to race. The heartrate increases periodically and the entire system begins to race. Hyperthyroidism is treatable, once treated wake sleep cycles should begin to return to normal.

Nasal and sinus allergies have symptoms that make it hard for a sufferer to sleep and stay asleep. Back drip from the sinus can interrupt sleep and blockage of nasal airways make it difficult to fall asleep and stay asleep.

Medication used to treat allergies and decongest the sinus and nasal cavities can also stimulate the system and make it difficult to sleep. Proper treatment can alleviate the symptoms and help restore normal sleep patterns.

Gastrointestinal problems can and do interrupt sleep. Acid reflux and other issues can keep sufferers awake and make it difficult for them to sleep through the night.

Neurological conditions can cause sleep disturbances and can also trigger insomnia. One neurological condition that can make it difficult to sleep is restless leg syndrome. Those with restless leg syndrome can experience the symptoms of this condition while trying to fall asleep or they may be jarred awake by the condition.

Each condition listed here can trigger insomnia, using the 7 steps without seeking treatment for these conditions will only ease the insomnia, no stop it. Treating these conditions will help resolve the insomnia and the 7 steps will eliminate it completely.

Chapter 3: Boost Your Day's Sleep

Although there are 24 hours in a day, most of them are already reserved for other activities that do not include restful sleeping. You often get tempted to work overtime or until after midnight even against your natural sleep patterns. But regardless of how hard it is to rest after each long day, be aware that each night's rest is a non-negotiable priority. You therefore must be efficient and use the 24 hours we have in a day to the best of your ability. This is the only way you can completely rest and refresh your bodily processes.

That said what should you do to ensure that you get a continuous cycle of high-quality sleep. The only guarantee to ensure that you sleep soundly is to maintain a friendly routine soon after you wake up, during the day and soon before you get to bed. Simply by devoting minimal time to the actual preparation of sleeping, while focusing primarily on getting quality sleep every night, you can get the rest you need to live the life you've always wanted with more energy and passion every day.

The following steps can help you perform better and still obtain sufficient sleep under a strict timeline:

When You Wake Up In The Morning

There are few measures that you can take to ensure you get quality sleep the night or day ahead. However, the most recommendable and effective strategy is to try sleeping in different phases. Scientists developed a concept referred to as Polyphasic sleep, where you simply break up your sleep into multiple short blocks as opposed to one long single block. For instance, you can choose to be biphasic sleeper in that you sleep shorter durations daily. You can decide to wake up at 8 AM, get into your schedule until lunch, get into another 2 hours nap, and continue to work until 2 AM. This concept also allows you to take 20-minute naps every 4 hours, though this can become complicated or difficult to follow.

To utilize sleep-in-phases concept, you only need to adapt flexible schedules that can help you get into regular nap routines that suit your working schedule. To develop one, be aware that good quality sleep shouldn't involve use of over the counter medication in order to influence your body's natural functions or senses. You don't have to force sleep or attempt to fall asleep more quickly, but it's a healthier thing to wake up easily, energized and feeling more refreshed.

If you rarely manage a minimum of 6 hours of sleep at night, a more recommendable routine is to take a 20-minute afternoon nap in your office. Try setting a timer for 20 minutes and then briefly lie on the couch with an eyeshade. Since taking medication isn't a good idea, try doing meditation or other mindfulness exercises such as repeating a single mantra as you inhale. For instance, you can choose a mantra like "happiness", "love", "peace" or pick other phrases that best describe you. With these steps, majority of people have managed to fall asleep and wake up naturally after 20 minutes even without a timer.

If you find napping in your office rather strange or unprofessional, you can inform your employees, work counterparts or other people that you'd take a longer period at the coffee outlet. However, this might not work always as per your script. Sometimes you may have to stay up late or probably awaken earlier by your kids. That's why you should follow a regular routine while in the office, or take naps in other random places such as in the car as you wait to pick your kid up. For example, you can take a 15 minutes nap at 8 AM as you drop kids to school, another short nap at 11 AM and later 15 minutes in the mid-afternoon.

The main idea is to get asleep as soon as you feel fatigued or tired as this helps you sleep faster and thus maximize productivity. There are times you'll need to work up the entire nights but you can find ways of extending your schedule. When very busy in the house, take 20-minute naps on your couch for every 2-4 hours, which should total to at least 1 hour of sleep time. With a 3-4 nap schedule, you can manage to work up overnight and still manage to wake up fresh and less tired, albeit for a few days.

● Be appreciative

One of the worst things about waking up early is the negative effect it has on your emotions. You wake up feeling groggy and grumpy and do not want to talk to anyone. It is important to take some time when you have just woken up to reflect on your life, otherwise you will go through the rest of the day with that ugly feeling. When you wake up in the morning, take some time to reflect on the things in your life. Give thanks for your work, your family, and friends in your life and realize how different your life would be without them; Be grateful for your wife or husband, for your kids, and for your boyfriend or girlfriend. Do this through meditation i.e.

take a few deep breaths, each time bringing into picture the person you are grateful for. Let this person sink in with every breath you take, then say a little prayer for the person; or just bless them. Simply being grateful puts your mind in a positive attitude. This attitude helps you wake up feeling nice and warm and motivates you throughout the day.

● Reward yourself

You might find that waking up early in the morning can be terribly dissatisfying because of the early morning drowsiness you experience. You sometimes wake up tired and even feel sleepy; sometimes, you end up giving up and falling back to bed. This is because you have not set the appropriate goals that will super boost you out of bed immediately that alarm clock starts to ring. Setting a reward for yourself when you wake up motivates you to get up and puts you in a better mood than waking up without any motivation. When you are motivated, you are likely to be more productive and enjoy your day than when you are not. It does not have to be a great deal per se, but just something to keep you going.

You can achieve other benefits with this strategy. Another great advantage of rewarding yourself in the morning is that it helps instill discipline needed to wake up early in the morning. When you know that there is a reward in waking up early, you do your best to go to bed as early as possible so that you wake up early. When you have accomplished your goal of waking up early throughout the month, you will be happy because of your achievements, and will even enjoy your reward happily. Here are a few ways you can reward yourself in the morning:

1. You can promise yourself a gift when you wake up at the exact time your alarm rings for the whole week.

2. You can put your coffee maker in your room. That way, you can reward yourself with a cup of coffee when you wake up to start your system.

3. Watching a morning show or news can also be a great source of motivation to get you started.

During The Day

There are also steps that you can undertake during the day to facilitate good sleep that day especially if you have a busy schedule. The worst thing is when the simple steps you want to take fail to make sense! For instance, sometimes after a busy day, you may need to take a few naps to relieve tiredness or tension but soon you become wide awake and frustrated.

The bad side is that lack of sleep during this stipulated period may cause involuntary sleep in the course of working time.

Nevertheless, you need to be creative here. Let's say you have a very busy schedule like strict deadlines to observe, tasks to perform and other demanding responsibilities. On the positive side, obtaining a 20-minute restful sleep can help rejuvenate you and calm your anxious mind. However, if you have a hard time sleeping during the mid-morning or afternoon break, you need to learn how to nap.

Different people may feel an urge to take the occasional nap anytime during the day. But the majority of people often feel like napping at around 3-5 PM when their energy levels have dropped. You need to take a couple of naps with each no longer than 20 minutes, as exceeding this time might leave you unsteady or unable to fall asleep later in bed. Knowing your sleep patterns can help you lighten the mood, boost your productivity, and feel better.

To understand your sleep patterns, keep a sleep diary to help you track your thoughts, daily habits and sleep patterns. It's easy to establish the time you go to bed, how long it takes to get a nap, whether you wake up before morning and when you wake up. This is very important for busy people and new moms who have an erratic sleep schedule. Experts advise people to avoid napping after 7 hours from getting up from bed. In case you feel sleepy, try napping early, but not 7 hours after waking up as this can mess your sleep routine. Such disruption can cause you to sleep late and thus wake up late as well.

In The Evening

Regardless of the amount of work or tiredness making you anxious, you have to get ready for a sweet and peaceful sleep. These few techniques can help you get prepared a few hours before getting to bed:

● Converse with yourself

The main factor that hinders effective sleep is stress. That's why you need to concentrate your mind to yourself in order to help drain stressors of life. Talk to yourself silently on topics that don't create stress. For instance, talk about what you'd like to carry on tonight. Also try to dialogue with your inner self about your dreams or aspirations.

● Play a game

Another way to calm down the mind is to play a few mindful games such as counting your breath. When in your office and unable to play games, take advantage of the rhythm and monotony of counting as this can soothe your mind. You can also count sheep, and focus on maintaining the sheep jumping a fence. The little level of concentration in this game can create enough stimulation to work up late or sleep better.

You can also choose to play real games, such as crossword puzzles or solitaire. For real games, place the game material where you can easily assess them, and under low light. I would recommend that you try out solitaire since the game is repetitive, not demanding and requires concentration with less mental effort. However, if you want to reduce screen time or avoid the blue light, playing the card version can help you relaxed compared to the computerized version under bright light.

During the Night

Do you want to start your day well in the morning? Then ensure that you get the right amount of sleep the night before. If you do not get enough sleep, you will wake up feeling tired, grumpy, and sleepy. The rest of your day will be less productive and you will be more vulnerable to accidents because of lack of concentration. When you have determined the right amount of sleep you need, create a routine so that you go to bed and wake up at the same time every day.

Train your brain to prepare to sleep by creating a sequence of habits before going to sleep. You can start by taking dinner, having a shower, reading a book, listening to some music and then going to bed. Here are a few steps to help you get enough sleep during the night:

● **Pray**

Different people have distinct beliefs. Regardless of your belief, it's important to say a little prayer before going to sleep. Praying helps to relax your mind by focusing and letting go of your worries. Prayer works in a similar way as meditation. If you do not pray when you go to sleep, are tensed, and worried, the stresses accumulated through the day can haunt you in your sleep. You will sleep uncomfortably because you are worried what tomorrow will be like.

Studies have shown that many cases revolving around insomnia are caused by stress. As such, when you pray, you put your mind to rest and forget the stresses affecting your life. Prayer can help you feel at peace right before you go to sleep. When you are praying, your mind relaxes and helps you let go of your day's worries and stresses, making it easier to sleep. You also enjoy a good night's sleep when you pray because you have faith that you are at peace and that nothing can scare you because you have a super natural being watching over you. This helps you to have a good night's sleep, free from nightmares and restlessness.

Thus, before you tuck yourself to sleep, make sure that you are in a state of peace and calm. If necessary, take out your spiritual book of your choice then read a few verses to help you meditate and relax. After reading the verses, keep calm and close your eyes to pray. Say a short prayer about the things affecting your life. Then you have to believe that all your problems are under control, and then jump to bed.

Majority of believers often report experiencing improved sleep after regular practice of prayers.

● Cool down:

Do you struggle to sleep and find yourself wriggling uncomfortably in your bed? This could be because of the temperature in your room. Being in a room that is either too hot or too cold makes it hard for your body to achieve the internal temperature set point that your brain is accustomed for you to fall asleep. For instance, high temperatures can affect you in several ways. For instance, you become sweaty or restless, and eventually wake up. Therefore, before going to sleep, achieve the ideal temperature for your room by following these simple guidelines:

1. Set the optimal temperature: The ideal temperature your room needs for a good

night's sleep is around 19-21 degrees Celsius. Adjust the thermostat in your air conditioner to meet that range. Getting your room to the temperature range of 19-21 degrees Celsius helps your body reach this temperature faster.

2. Allow Air in the house: On a hot day, close the curtains and blinds to prevent sunlight, and open them when the sun is setting. Open the windows too to let in that cool evening breeze into your room.

3. Install a fan to help maintain the room cool. The general idea is to make your room cooler so that your body reaches the set point temperature faster. Getting a fan helps to eliminate excess heat that may make it uncomfortable to sleep.

● **Relax**

To get a good night sleep, it's vital for you to be relaxed. Keeping your mind at rest is the key to getting a good night's sleep. Being prepared to sleep helps your mind get rid of any disturbances, especially by taking big breaths and visualizing. When you are in a relaxed state, your mind takes time to slowly take in the day's activities and consolidate any new things learnt without tension. This way, you are able to enjoy a good night's sleep and wake up feeling refreshed in the morning that follows.

On the other hand, when you are not relaxed before going to bed, chances are high that you will not get a good night's sleep. You will be restless at night, twisting and turning before you go to sleep. Your dreams can also be affected if you go to sleep when you are tensed; or worse still experience nightmares in your sleep! Here are a few steps to help you out:

1. Stop doing any work at least one hour before going to bed to help your mind settle before sleeping.

2. Use some breathing techniques outlined here to help you relax. Take a few breaths, hold your abdomen and chest for a while, and then breathe out. Repeat this exercise a few times.

3. Train your brain to sleep with a sleeping routine. Set a specific time to go to bed as well as waking up.

4. Make your room as comfortable as possible. Let your brain know that your room is meant for sleeping and sex only by getting rid of any work related materials on your bed. Let it be dark by turning off all the lights.

5. You can take advantage of your diary, or just a small notebook to write down the things that happened that day, your

achievements and so on. This will help to clear your mind and obtain relaxation.

6. Write down any problem that may be causing tension in your life now. Also write any possible solutions on the same paper and then throw it away with your tension.

7. Visualize: imagine you are in a place of peace and tranquility. Use your senses to feel the place and consequently relax your mind.

Note: While what we've covered so far is very helpful in getting you to sleep, you can still benefit a lot more by learning some more specifics that will get you to sleep without trouble. Let's discuss this in detail in the subsequent chapters.

Chapter 4: Understanding Sleep Apnea

One common sleeping disorder is called sleep apnea. This is when a person can never achieve a sound sleep because they are constantly waking up during the night. The scary part of this disorder is that several times a night the sufferer actually stops breathing for a short amount of time and then restarts as they wake up. There is no memory of the fact that they stop breathing and to the individual they believe that they are sleeping through the night. The symptoms will be chronic fatigue, unexplained irritability and a lack of productivity during the day. Some suffers will constantly doze off when given the opportunity during the day. They could be sitting in a chair talking to you one minute and then snoring the next and jumping right back into the conversation the next. This disease is particularly dangerous and can cause serious health issues.

Sleep Apnea is a potentially life threatening ailment because of the long term physical effects and stress that the constant lack of sound sleep brings to a person. If there is a suspicion of sleep apnea a person should see a doctor right away so that one of many different treatment options can be implemented. This is a sleep ailment that can be cured and getting rid of the constant fatigue and tiredness will allow a person to take back their life.

The level of sleep apnea will determine what type of measures a person will have to take. For the most serious cases there are sleep centers that specialize in treating many sleep ailments as well as sleep apnea. This is for the most serious cases. Another cure is to take continuous positive airway pressure, (CPAP). This method has a mask like device fitted over the face of the sleeping patient steaming air into the patient continuously while they sleep. It prevents the person from the stressful breathing stops that cause such damage to a person. It can be difficult to become comfortable wearing the sleep apnea mask and listening to he machine that constantly pumps the air into your body. However the lack of comfort is much better than not sleeping at all and eventually experiencing death.

For mild to moderate cases of the infliction the cures are a lot easier. Sometimes simply sleeping in a different position can allow a person to breath better through the night. For many people, the cure can be as simple as losing some excess weight. Unfortunately, the easy cures won't work for a lot of people.

Chapter 5: Sleep Apnea And Surgery

Having a surgical procedure for Sleep Apnea may seem like a quick remedy, but one needs to look at the risks involved too. If a person is already suffering from ailments such as high blood pressure, diabetes or heart disease, the surgery can only be performed after analyzing the level of risk these ailments could cause. Such decisions cannot be taken overnight.

The surgeon may need some time to analyze these factors and figure out whether it is safe for you to undergo surgery or not. This is critical when it comes to performing surgeries on small children.

A surgery for Sleep Apnea issues should only be considered after you have exhausted all other treatment options.

This could also mean that you would need to remove your tonsils or adenolds. Before going down the path for surgery, the following tests would need to be conducted by your doctor.

☐ Tests for other ailments (blood pressure, blood sugar, heart diseases)

☐ X-ray

☐ CT Scan

☐ Blood test

Types of Surgeries for Sleep Apnea problems

a) Nasal Surgery

Chronic nasal congestion is one of the primary reasons why patients may opt for surgery. Nasal obstructions affect the turbinate, septum and the nasal tract, which further increase the Sleep Apnea issues. If you have tried everything to cure your chronic nasal congestion and nothing seems to fix the problem, you may need to consider getting nasal surgery.

Turbinate reduction is typically performed in these cases and is well received by most people. It involves less risk than the other surgeries. The surgery, once performed, can unclog the airway, allowing easier flow of air.

In people who suffer from a valve collapse due to a fragile lower nose cartilage, the septum can be positioned to increase their strength.

These procedures can be carried out without much hassle and the person tends to recover quickly.

b) Soft Palate Implants

Soft Palate implant procedures are also known as "pillar procedures" that can be used to treat Sleep Apnea problems. It is widely used nowadays and can be performed in just a few hours. This surgery requires placing 3 polyester rods in the soft palate, which activate the inflammatory reaction of the soft tissues around it.

This could strengthen the tissues, which in turn will minimize the contact with the rear pharynx wall and gradually reduce Sleep Apnea. This surgery is so simple that it can be performed by your local doctor, with or without anesthesia.

c) Tongue enhancement surgery

In this procedure, the genioglossus muscles of the tongue are enhanced in order to keep the tongue from lying backwards while the patient is sleeping.

This procedure involves making a slight cut in the jaw bone, removing it and attaching it back with a short titanium disc, which can prevent the tongue from falling backwards.

It is an extensive surgery and uses a lot of advanced techniques. The person would need to be admitted for at least 24 hours in the hospital, and is kept under observation for a few hours after the surgery. A lot of doctors may use this technique only if the Sleep Apnea problem is severe in an individual.

d) Tongue lower base reduction

The lower base of the tongue is found to be one of the reasons why people with Sleep Apnea experience aggravated symptoms. Tongue base reduction can be done using various advanced techniques, to correct Apnea problems in people. The radio frequency wave technique is preferred by most doctors, as it has shown positive results in people, more than most other surgeries.

It positions the radio frequency waves to particular zones in the tongue without causing any harm to other tissue. This surgery is not too time consuming and the person can be discharged within a day of performing this operation. A general anesthesia is enough to help a person to tolerate the pain during the surgical procedure.

e) Jaw enhancement

Narrow or smaller jaws can restrict airflow and impact Sleep Apnea patients to a larger extent. A Maxillomandibular enhancement is recommended in such patients, and can help enhance the upper airway by extending the jaw frame. For this, the upper and lower jaw bones are fitted with titanium plates by making a precise cut in the jaw bones.

This is a very difficult surgery that should only be performed by an expert. One needs to pick the right surgeon, as this procedure is very complex. It is also a very painful procedure that requires a person to be completely sedated with anesthesia during the process.

The person is required to stay in the hospital for 24-48 hours after the surgery and can only be discharged once he/she completely recovers. The teeth need to be secured using wire and only liquid food can be consumed to prevent putting pressure on the jaws.

f) Tracheotomy

Tracheotomy is performed to create an entrance in the neck of the patient that paves the way for straight access to the trachea. This type of surgical procedure is performed only on patients who are seriously ill, or during emergencies. There is a possibility of serious complications occurring that could further complicate matters. Nevertheless, it is a highly effective surgery, which can cure the Sleep Apnea problem in a patient, completely and quickly. There are a few ill-effects that are experienced by some patients post surgery. They are listed as below:

If the surgical procedure is not performed properly, a correction surgery may be needed to fix the larynx or airway.

In some people, this operation can trigger numerous allergies or even an infection.

An inappropriately performed operation can lead to scarring of the airway.

Although it is rare, a tracheotomy may result in excessive blood loss and require a blood transfusion.

The throat can hurt for a while post surgery, making it difficult to swallow solid food. However, this problem typically goes away after a few days on by itself.

g) Hyoid Enhancement Surgery

Hyoid suspension is an excellent cure for Sleep Apnea. This procedure aims at relieving Apnea issues by clearing the obstructed airway. It requires that a slight suture be inserted below the chin to aid the tongue. The hyoid bone is located in the tongue where the pharynx and tongue muscles are connected.

Since the tongue often falls backwards while sleeping, it often makes contact with the pharynx wall and disrupts the airflow. This operation requires two incisions to be made on the neck. The surgery can be completed within a few minutes and the person can be discharged almost immediately. There are typically no side-effects or pain post-surgery. Since it helps them recover faster, more people feel open to this type of surgery.

Chapter 6: Sleep Disorders & Related Conditions

It may well be the case that you have made an assessment of your situation and you think that you might have an underlying sleep related condition. This book is not a medical resource as such, however it is useful to give an introduction to some of the most common sleep disorders and diseases. It stands to reason that if you think you may be affected by any of these, or you have wider issues relating to sleep, then a visit to your doctor is an excellent course of action to follow. Some of the hints and tips later in this book may help however, and you may want to give them a go. Common sleep related disorders and conditions then, include:

Insomnia is difficulty getting to sleep in the first place, or when you manage to, staying asleep for long enough to feel refreshed the next morning - even if you have had enough opportunity to sleep. It is estimated that insomnia can affect around one in three of the population at certain times. It is quite a wide definition, and is so quite common. With insomnia you can find it difficult to nod off in the first place, or you may find yourself waking through the night, and lying awake. It may be that you wake at a certain time, perhaps early in the morning, and cannot get back to sleep. Related to this is not feeling refreshed when you get yourself up in the morning. You may also find it tricky to nap during the day. Insomnia can have many underlying sources – for example stress or anxiety, unsuitable sleeping environment, factors relating to lifestyle (diet, drinking, jet lag, shift work), mental health conditions, physical health conditions and certain medicines. Some of these factors are considered elsewhere in this book, but in addition you may wish to consider trying to relax before bedtime, and trying to set regular times for going to bed and waking up. This is a condition where your doctor may also be able to suggest some possibilities (which can even include cognitive therapy).

Body clock disorders – as we have discussed our bodies respond to a circadian rhythm. Where your body does not quite configure with a typical rhythm, this can be known as circadian rhythm sleep disorder. There are a number of conditions under this umbrella. For example delayed phase sleep disorder means that whilst someone can show a normal length and quality of sleep, this takes place later than most people – so, for example, falling asleep at three in the morning rather than eleven o'clock the previous evening. There are other circadian rhythm disorders, such as Non-24 which is when an individual can have a hard time sleeping at night, but has a strong urge to nap at other times. Common in people who are completely blind, Non-24 is a result of the master body clock running slightly longer than 24 hours. Whilst this happens for most people, with this disorder, that extra time adds up, causing a noticeable change in sleeping rhythms. This is a relatively little researched disorder, and the first step is to talk to your doctor about the issue - but be aware that not all clinicians may be up to speed with the condition. There are support groups who can arm you with some facts before you meet your doctor.

Snoring

Snoring is extremely common, and is effectively just noisy breathing during sleep. Whilst that might be easy to say, it can have a serious effect on the sleep of the person snoring, and anyone who might happen to be sharing a bed (or a house in extreme cases) with them. It is more common in males, and being overweight can exacerbate the problem. Snoring can also show itself more as an individual gets older. Some people who sleep loudly also suffer from other conditions, such as sleep apnea (discussed later). When you sleep, many of your body's muscles relax. This is exactly the same for your throat and tongue, where the walls of the throat vibrate gently when you breathe in, and sometimes when you breathe out too – this is what causes the sound. There are reasons why snoring can become worse. These include the ageing process (where the throat muscles relax more) or abnormalities in the nose or throat. Even sleeping position (usually on the back) can cause snoring – that one can be relatively easily rectified, especially if accompanied by a reminder from someone you may be close to. Many snorers do not realise they are doing it, so it might be that someone else tells you before you appreciate there is a problem. Some of the lifestyle changes we refer to later can help, but surgery for certain conditions is also an option. There are a variety of devices on the market to try and alleviate snoring – some of these are fitted by dentists or other professionals but others can be more self-help tools. One of the most recent on the market even uses headphone style noise reduction technology to counter the noise of the snoring. If you or a friend / family member is concerned about your snoring, go and see a doctor.

Breathing disorders

The condition sleep apnea was mentioned earlier – effectively this is where there is a cessation of breathing as the walls of the throat relax too much – this requires medical attention as it can be very serious, and is sometimes treated by the wearing of kit which prevents the back of the throat from collapse – this should only be prescribed by a qualified doctor.

Movement disorders

Periodic Limb Movements in Sleep – this is movement, repetitive in nature, which sees brief muscle twitches or jerking – most likely related to the nervous system. As with many sleep conditions, this is likely to be of most irritation to anyone else sleeping in the bed, and is not considered to be a serious condition but if it is having a big impact, speak to a medical professional..

Restless Legs Syndrome – this syndrome is experienced by a surprisingly large number of people — estimated at ten percent of the American population. The syndrome is categorised by an urge to move legs when at rest, often accompanied by unpleasant sensations. This can affect individuals through the day, but can have particular effects at night. It can be treated, through active management of lifestyle, though it can be that treatment of veins in legs can make a difference — again, one for you to talk through with your doctor.

Teeth Grinding — this is another common condition, but it can have effects such as dental damage, pain in the facial muscles and can lead to headaches. It is thought this can be worse when sleeping on your back, and may also be linked to daytime stress or sleep deprivation. In severe cases dentists may prescribe a soft bespoke appliance — but this would be for a professional to dictate.

Medical conditions

Attention deficit/hyperactivity disorder, or ADHD, describes activity which results in inattentiveness and behaviour based on impulse. It begins in childhood, but can persist through adulthood – children with the disorder often need particular support from those around them, and healthcare/schooling systems. ADHD has been linked with a number of sleep related issues. Whilst adults tend to become sluggish when tired, children can show the opposite behaviour – this means that a child not getting enough sleep can be confused with having ADHD. Medication can help control some of the systems, though there are side effects. Other recommended considerations include social skills training, psychotherapy (therapy used to treat emotional or mental health problems) and support in relation to behaviours. Stable household regimes, and a relaxing bedtime routine may also help, and it is recommended that ADHD children get sufficient exercise every day.

Alzheimer's disease affects cognitive abilities, and the ability to carry out everyday activities. The disease does affect sleep, and it is considered that patients will experience disrupted sleep - this will vary individual to individual, and on the stage of the disease. Sleep problems and agitation can lead to stress for those giving care. Whilst there is no known cure for the disease, there are medicinal and behavioural therapies which can slow its effects. This is a complex condition, and it is highly recommended that carers get support. However there are some recommended aids – these include trying to get some form of exercise every day, creating a relaxed sleep environment (as discussed elsewhere), having an evening and sleep routine, and getting into brighter light soon after waking in the morning. Dementia, describes a group of symptoms, the most common cause of which is Alzheimer's disease.

Asthma is a common condition affecting the lungs, and sufferers often experience disrupted sleep as a result of coughing and breathlessness. Some researchers believe there is a link between asthma and the circadian rhythms (though not all asthma sufferers experience such night time symptoms. It is thought that at the onset of sleep, asthma sufferers can have a good airway function, which can decrease the longer an individual sleeps. In addition, there are a wide variety of factors which can lead to an asthma attack. These include colds, smoke, dust mites and even weather – asthma support groups and online resources should be able to help you identify the triggers which most affect you. Asthma cannot be cured, but can be medically controlled – however these are for discussion with a medical professional. Actions you can take at home include those factors relating to a good bedtime environment and regime discussed elsewhere.

Chronic obstructive pulmonary disease, or COPD, describes chronic lung disorders such as bronchitis or emphysema. Those with such conditions may find that a change in breathing patterns can lead to a reduction in blood oxygen. Smoking can be a key cause, and so it makes sense to try and stop this to try and reduce symptoms. There are also drug and behavioural therapies which can help, and patients can be prescribed oxygen. Measures for a healthy sleep environment are very important for this condition, though you will also want to talk to your doctor about any medical options. The wider picture is important with this sort of condition, so give thought to your diet and exercise options – again discuss with your doctor.

Depression – feeling sad at certain times of our lives is part of the gambit of human emotions – however where such feeling persist, or include anxiety, a feeling of hopelessness and disinterest, then this could be diagnosed as depression. This is an extremely common condition, and its relationship with sleep can be complex. It may be that depression causes sleep issues, or it may be the other way around, that sleep issues can contribute to depression. Whilst these issues can be discussed with trained professionals, we have talked elsewhere about what can potentially be done for the sleep problems themselves. You may find that actions taken to improve sleep (relaxing bedtime routine, reducing clutter) may help with both depression and your sleep issues. It is not being suggested that things are necessarily that simple however, and it is recommended that you speak to your doctor or one of the depression support groups out there – this is important as the condition can be as individual as you – and bespoke arrangements will help you best. For some people the condition seasonal affective disorder (SAD) can be an issue – this sees circadian rhythms becoming mixed up as the days get shorter in winter, and this can trigger depression – this tends to be resolved in springtime, but there can be light related measures taken through the winter. There are a variety of medicinal and behavioural options available to treat depression, but these should be discussed with an individual trained in these matters – it might be useful to build an analysis of your mood into a diary – which of course can include exercise, diet and sleep patterns too.

Epilepsy is a condition which can result in seizures (or convulsions). Other conditions can cause such reactions, however those with epilepsy often have other issues to deal with, such as social problems. Epilepsy, however, can be controlled, and most patients are able to lead active and long lives. Epilepsy can disturb sleep, and sleep deprivation can trigger seizures. This means that wider consideration of your sleep environment is critical. If you live with someone who has epilepsy, then your sleep pattern can affect their condition too – so you may have to make some changes too. As with other conditions, medical treatment is for discussion with a doctor, but it may be possible to work in some alternative therapies too. Epilepsy support groups should be able to help with useful possibilities – as well as giving the proper advice on what to do if someone is having a seizure.

Acid reflux, or gastroesophagael reflux disease (GERD) is relatively common and can lead to night time heartburn – which not surprisingly can affect sleep patterns. Effectively this condition sees a backflow of acid from the gut, and symptoms can be worse when sleeping or trying to sleep. Certain foods are associated with reflux – it might be worth keeping a food and sleep diary if you are affected. Some recommendations include avoiding lying down after a large meal, eating smaller portions and trying to have an upright posture. Medical treatments are available, and you should consult your doctor about the options.

Multiple Sclerosis (MS) is a condition affecting the immune system. It can have some severe symptoms, but can be managed to allow patients to have fulfilling and active lives. MS is associated with sleep disorders including insomnia and nocturnal leg spasms. MS can lead to issues related to vision, muscle, senses and balance, as well as sleep disorders. As a complex condition, diagnosis and treatment is for healthcare professionals, but given that a good sleep can alleviate some symptoms, it is important to consider this – and to see whether the wider improvements to bed environment and routine might help. There are also medicinal and behavioural options relating to sleep – talk to your doctor about the options. Alternative therapies may also work for you, and support groups may be able to help with ideas.

Sudden Infant Death Syndrome (SIDS) is the sudden and unexpected death of an infant less than one year old, who had appeared healthy immediately before the death. Of course this is an incredibly traumatic event, and it is one that it has been suggested has a peak risk point of two to three months old, and in the USA has higher incidences in African American or Native American populations than in Caucasians. Incidences have declined through the 1990s, 2000s and 2010s – largely attributed to campaigns to have babies and infants sleep on their backs. Whilst there are a number of researched medical theories considered relevant to the condition, there are also a number of behavioural factors which can increase the possibility of the Syndrome. These can include: the infant sleeping on their stomach; the use of soft bedding or unsafe beds (for example couches or waterbeds); loose bedding materials (blankets, pillows), overheating (clothing or room temperature); mother's age younger than 20 years old; mother smoking during pregnancy (or exposure to secondhand smoke); mother receiving late or no prenatal care; premature birth or low weight birth. It is advisable to consult with professional bodies with detailed information on this issue, some of which also point to some myths around the issue – for example that immunizations can be a cause; that side sleeping is as safe as back sleeping (it isn't – infants can roll onto their stomachs); infants are at greater risk of choking on their backs (doctors have not found this); and sleeping on the back flattens the back of the head (any such flat spot tends to go away once the child is sitting up). The impact of a SIDS event can be traumatic for others in the family, and can affect sleep overall – it is well worth seeking professional support at such a traumatic time.

Other conditions and disorders

Nightmares – these are dreams which can affect children and adults alike, though are perhaps more common in children. A nightmare can feel very realistic, and can contain some content which is worrying. In addition, nightmares tend to be recalled well.

REM behaviour disorder – whilst dreaming is primarily something experienced in the brain, those who suffer from REM behaviour disorder find themselves acting out their dreams. This can involve physical movements during the dreaming phase of sleep – in some circumstances this can lead to danger for the individual, or others around them – on some cases it can include sleep talking or sleep walking.

Sleepwalking – though often described as sleepwalking, actually this condition can see individuals carrying out some tasks – though more often they can be sitting up in bed, or walking around a room or house – all whilst in a deep sleep. This is a relatively common occurrence, though more so in children. Sleepwalkers are often difficult to wake up, and it might even be that they engage in some unusual behaviour, such as going to the toilet in places other than the bathroom.

Sleep talking – talking in sleep can take the form of incoherent speech, or it can be much more coherent. The individual will not know that they are talking at the time – but others might and this can lead to more general sleep disruption. If sleep talking is a real issue or continues over a long period of time, then consider the wider aids to sleep covered elsewhere in this book. It may be that some of these factors would improve overall sleep quality, and cut down on sleep talking.

Bedwetting – Whilst wetting the bed can be fairly common for young children going through potty training, it is not uncommon in children up to the age of seven.

Bedwetting after a period of bladder control through the night may be linked to an underlying condition, or psychological stress. It can happen occasionally uo to the age of five or so, but if it happens more regularly after that it might be worth a trip to the doctor. It is worth making sure your child goes to the bathroom just before bedtime and if you can combine this with a good and consistent bedtime routine, then the results may be positive. It might also be worth lifting your child to go to the bathroom before you go to bed – and before they might wet the bed. Of course it makes sense to avoid late night drinks. Reward systems such as stickers for a dry bed, and positive words around how good it is for them to have made it through the night dry are a good plan. In extreme cases a doctor may prescribe medication. There are other possible measures you can utilise to save on damage – these include duvet and sleeping bag liners – and if required, absorbent underpants – though these are not for long term use. Try not to be angry with children who wet the bed – work with them to get through it, and they won't learn to dread bed and going to sleep.

Daytime sleepiness disorders – such disorders mean that individuals can feel tired, even if they have had a good night of sleep. It might be that you feel excessively tired through the day due to an underlying condition – such as those we have explored earlier. Another symptom to consider is, if you find that you are getting plenty of sleep, and find yourself also falling asleep through the day, then that, too, can be a warning sign. Some people have the condition narcolepsy – this is where an individual will, overall, not sleep any more than another individual, but cannot control when that sleep might take place. In addition, an individual might have this accompanied by a condition which can see them lose muscle control and have some other sleep disorder symptoms when asleep. Obviously this is a dangerous condition, and requires, at least, medical evaluation – treatments can include medication, together with action on behaviour. Occasional short naps can help, as can some of the wider measures discussed elsewhere.

Finally, you may want to be aware of hormone changes – these are natural changes which can take place which affect things like the temperature of an individual, how they feel more generally in feeling comfortable to sleep, and the need to urinate through the night. Such hormone changes can take place through pregnancy and the menopause. For women who are pregnant, a mix of comfortable clothing, and pillows for

support as you grow larger can help —
experiment with the pillows for your most
comfortable position. Hormone changes
through the menopause can lead to
overheating — again comfortable, light
clothes and keeping your room cool can
help.

Chapter 7: Devices And Surgery As Aids

For those with severe sleep apnea issues and the lack of time to properly embark on a natural course of cure, there is also the faster and easier route to a solution while you practice the slower and more permanent route. These tools are here to get you quick relief, but remember to make lifestyle changes and to follow some of the exercises listed in the last chapter.

As you saw in the earlier chapters, there are three distinct categories of sleep apnea. The mechanical devices here are not all suitable for all the different types. If the problem is physical, meaning it is OSA, the devices will offer the best relief. If however the problem is more towards a defect in the CNS, then the devices will not be too much help and you will need other remedies listed in the next chapter.

CPAP for Sleep Apnea

Known as the most common treatment for both moderate and severe cases of OSA, CPAP or Continuous Positive Airflow Pressure involves the use of a mask-like machine providing a continuous stream of air. This helps breathing passages open.

CPAP provides a compressor that is placed close to the bed and a hose that straps to a mask worn around the head. That mask from a semi tight seal, which then transmits air from the pump to the nose under pressure. The pressurized air then keeps the passages in the body open. The increased pressure also increases the oxygen diffusion there by increasing the pulse oxygen levels. The positive pressure environment in the airways allows the breathing to continue smoothly and sleep is not distracted. This is obviously a fix for OSA and not CSA.

Just note that the CPAP can be uncomfortable to don and many patients find it a nuisance at night.

Tips for Adjusting to a CPAP Unit

First, check for proper fit. If the mask is snug, it will be a lot easier to wear through the night. If the mask is too tight, it will be uncomfortable. It takes time to find the right fit.

Second, give yourself some time to get used to it. You will notice that the discomfort level is worth the increased sleep. You do not have to force yourself to like wearing the mask. Again, it is okay to feel weird about having to wear a mask to sleep. Start by wearing it for only short periods throughout the day.

Third, customize the device. Components of the CPAP machine including the straps, mask and the tubing can be customized to provide you with the best fit possible. There are also available soft pads. These pads can help in reducing skin irritation as a result of wearing the device. You can also get nasal pillows and chinstraps, which may help, lessen the chances of throat irritation.

Fourth, use it with a humidifier. A special moisturizer may also be applied before going to bed. In fact, latest models of CPAP are now equipped with a built-in humidifier.

Other Breathing Devices Recommended for Sleep Apnea

Sleep specialists may also recommend other breathing devices. Such recommendations may include Bilevel

Positive Airway Pressure (BPAP) and Adaptive Servo-Ventilation (ASV).

BPAP or Bilevel Positive Airway Pressure

This can be used as an alternative option to CPAP especially or patients who find it difficult to adjust to the CPAP unit.

The BPAP is designed to adjust the air pressure automatically as the patient sleeps. When the patient inhales, the device provides more pressure. And when you (the patient) exhales, the device adjusts and provides less air pressure. There are BPAP devices that are designed to help the patient breathe again when the unit detects the patient has not taken a breath for several seconds.

The BPAP is a sound alternative for those suffering with CSA. Because, in CSA the mind stops instructing the breathing muscles to perform, the BPAP continues to force air into the lungs, under the necessary pressure. It's like a ventilating machine that detects if the patient is breathing or otherwise then provides the air to compensate.

ASV or Adaptive Servo-Ventilation

Targeted for individuals with central and obstructive sleep apnea, ASV devices can monitor and store information about the patient's normal breathing pattern. It delivers airflow pressure, which is meant to prevent breathing pauses, which is one of the potentially dangerous symptoms of the condition.

Oral Appliances for Sleep Apnea

Dental devices are oral appliances that are recommended in place of CPAP and other devices. These appliances are more static as they fit on the mouth of the person and then stay that. It is like using braces on the teeth that adjust the positioning of the dental profile. They are not actively moving, but are there constantly applying pressure to adjust the shape.

For OSA, these devices are designed to keep the throat open as the throat has the tendency to relax and a relaxed throat can result in apnea. There are different designs for oral appliances. Some are engineered to bring the jaw forward. This mechanism can help with keeping the throat open. While oral appliances may be effective, they may not be as reliable as CPAP machines.

Most of these devices are made of acrylic. They can fit inside the mouth like a mouth guard that most athletes wear. There are other devices that can fit in the head and chin. Two of the most common dental devices available today are the tongue retaining and the mandibular repositioning device.

The main goal of these equipments is to bring the tongue and the lower jaw forward keeping the air passage open during sleep. They work by improving the tongue's muscle tone and repositioning the tongue, lower jaw, uvula and soft palate.

Oral appliances are simply more comfortable than the heavier and more cumbersome devices like the CPAP. It does not take a lot of time to get used to wearing these devices as compared to CPAP, which may take several months of adjustment. Just a couple of weeks to get used to it will suffice. Because these oral appliances are small, they are also convenient to carry.

Typically prescribed for mild and moderate cases of sleep apnea, dental devices may cause certain side effects, such as nausea, soreness, saliva buildup and mouth odor.

Surgical Procedures for Sleep Apnea

Surgery is always regarded as the last resort. Surgical procedures should only be considered after exhausting all other treatment options. Surgery may be performed to enlarge the size of the airway, which can reduce the occurrence of sleep apnea episodes.

Here are some procedures:

Shrinking

In cases of patients with abnormally enlarged airway, shrinking procedures may be performed. Somnoplasty for instance, makes use of radio frequency ablation in shrinking the soft palate, turbinates of the nose, base of the tongue and uvula.

Stiffening

Stiffening procedures are commonly performed through implants. It may be appropriate for sleep apneics who have soft palate that tends to interrupt with the airway. These implants are usually made of plastic and they are usually inserted or injected to the back of the mouth or in the soft palate.

Repositioning and Removal

Other procedures involve the removal of adenoids, tonsils or any excess tissue located either inside the nose or at the back of the throat. Repositioning procedures may also be performed. For instance, the jaw may be repositioned or reconstructed to increase space for the upper airway.

Before you consider surgery, make sure you are well informed about the procedure. Take note of the things you should expect. Keep in mind too that surgery usually comes with certain risks and complications. There is always a possibility of infection. But if you choose your surgeon carefully and you take good care of yourself before and after the procedure, you significantly lessen your risks.

Chapter 8: Diet-Related Factors

Caffeine: This is a powerful nervous system stimulant usually found in tea, coffee, chocolate, and sodas.

Point 1: There is a point where the body normally settles down to a restive mode when certain levels of adenosine are reached. Coffee works by filling up receptor sites meant for adenosine. Instead of feeling tired, the body just keeps on going because it is not getting the appropriate cues that allow it to rest and recover.

Point 2: The effects of caffeine are felt by the body even after five to eight hours after consumption.

Sleep Solution Tip:

Avoid caffeine consumption after two o'clock in the afternoon to ensure that the body has completely removed it from its systems before bedtime.

Magnesium: This mineral is known to have stress reducing properties. Its sleep-related functions include relaxing tensed muscles and calming the nervous system.

Point 1: Research has shown that one of the symptoms of magnesium deficiency is chronic insomnia or difficulty in getting to sleep.

Point 2: The most effective way of boosting up magnesium levels in the body is through the topical application of the mineral on the skin.

Sleep Solution Tips:

Include magnesium-rich foods in the diet such as:

Green leafy vegetables

Pumpkin seeds

Sesame seeds

Spirulina

Brazil nuts

Taking a bath in Epsom salts can help in the transdermal absorption of magnesium. Other topical forms of magnesium include magnesium bath flakes and magnesium oils.

The best places to apply topical magnesium are:

Anywhere in the body that is sore

On the chest

Around the neck and shoulders

Alcohol consumption: Drinking alcohol late in the evening will make a person fall asleep faster but the quality of sleep is severely compromised.

Point 1: With alcohol in its systems, the body is not able to fall into deeper levels of sleep.

Point 2: One of the most common sleep interruptions that arise from alcohol consumption is the need to pass urine. Every time a person wakes from an alcohol-induced sleep, it can be difficult to go back to sleep.

Sleep Solution Tips:

Avoid drinking alcohol at least four hours before going to bed.

Drinking water can help to nullify the effects of alcohol and help to flush it out faster.

Sleep Inducing Supplements:

1. Chamomile: This is an herb that is capable of helping to calm the nervous system and of making muscles relax.

2. Kava kava: This is a drink that originated from Fiji and has sedative properties. It is most often used to treat cases of insomnia and fatigue. It has properties that contribute to the improvement of sleep quality and to the decrease in the amount of time it takes to sleep.

3. Valerian: This herb is a moderate sedative that is indicated for use by people who a difficult time falling asleep. It is also known to promote uninterrupted sleep.

4. 5-HTP: This is a neurotransmitter that is a precursor to serotonin, which plays a role in the process of the sleep cycle. Studies have shown that people who took

5-HTP went to sleep faster and were able to sleep more deeply.

5. GABA: This is the major inhibitory neurotransmitter of the brain and as such plays an important role in inducing sleep. It is able to block the actions of excitatory brain chemicals allowing the brain to settle down and rest.

6. L-Tryptophan: This substance is the precursor to 5-HTP which was previously mentioned. Food sources include: turkey, chicken, pumpkin, sunflower seeds, and collard greens

7. Melatonin: Melatonin is effective as a sleep-inducing supplement but the downside is that it can interfere with the body's natural ability to produce its own melatonin. Furthermore, most hormonal therapies such as this come with a host of

side effects and potential health-related problems.

Side Effects:

irritability

dizziness

migraines

constipation

stomach pain

weight gain

Sleep Solution Tip:

Supplements give the most benefit when used in within a short time period to normalize sleeping patterns that have been temporarily disrupted such as during travel.

Some Night Snacking Sleep Solution Tips:

If you experience hunger pangs before bedtime, it is better to eat a high-fat, low-carbohydrate snack to keep the blood sugar stable and to avoid sugar crashes that might potentially disrupt sleep.

Allot ninety minute or more after eating before going to sleep.

Chapter 9: How To Diagnose Sleep Apnea With Sleep Studies

Sleep studies are generally carried out in a sleep center or a sleep laboratory. This might or might not be in a medical facility. If the study is performed in the sleep center, you might have an overnight stay. Nevertheless, this is not always engraved in stone.

The beneficial thing about sleep studies is that you will not endure any discomfort. The only thing that might impact you is skin irritation from the sensors. When the sensing units are removed from your skin, you will not deal with any more irritation.

Although the risks of sleep studies are marginal, these studies take some time (at least a couple of hours).

There are various tests for sleep studies. One of them is referred to as a polysomnogram or PSG test. This test is performed in a sleep center or sleep laboratory. More than likely, with this test, an overnight stay will be required.

You are going to have electrodes and monitors on your scalp, face, chest, limbs and fingers. As you are sleeping, the following things are going to be monitored:

- The motion of your eyes

- The activity in your brain

- The activity in your muscles

- The pace of your heart

- The tempo of your heart

- Blood pressure

- Air motion in and out of your lungs

- How much oxygen is in your blood

As you sleep, the staff on duty are going to utilize sensors to examine your as you sleep throughout the night. After the PSG is done, the sleep expert is going to go over the results with you. They are going to have the ability to identify whether you have sleep apnea and if it is serious or not. From the results, they are going to have the ability to chart a course of treatment.

A Multiple Sleep Latency Test or MSLT is utilized to identify how drowsy you are in the daytime. This test is generally carried out after a PSG. You will have devices put on your scalp for monitoring reasons.

With this test, you are going to need to take at least 5 naps, each lasting 20 minutes. This is supposed to be carried out every 2 hours throughout times when you would be alert. The testers are going to examine how long it is going to take you to go to sleep and how long you slept.

Those individuals who take less than 5 minutes to get to sleep are more likely prospects for a sleep disorder. When the screening is carried out, the sleep specialist is going to supply you with the results and talk to you about treatment options.

Where To Locate A Sleep Specialist

If you require help discovering a sleep specialist, there are a number of organizations that can help you with that, like:

- American Academy of Sleep Medicine (AASM)

- American Board of Sleep Medicine (ABSM)

- American Academy of Dental Sleep Medicine (AADSM)

These organizations are comprised of doctors, scientists and dentists that work with individuals impacted with this sleep disorder. They work to further the development of sleep medicine and sleep research.

The doctors and researchers that serve on the relevant boards are noted as "Board Certified" in the niche of sleep medicine. The ABSM keeps an updated listing of sleep specialists. They could be found by the state or by their name. The AADSM keeps an updated listing of dentists that focus on dealing with sleep apnea patients by utilizing oral devices.

Chapter 10: How A Little Movement Each Day Can Help You Sleep Better At Night

In Chapter Three, I talked about the need to set a bedtime ritual to help you sleep. I also mentioned that I do yoga as part of my own nighttime routine but that is not the only exercise that I get through the day. Exercise has now become as much of a part of my daily routine as going to work or eating meals. It is something that I look forward to. It is something that is very important for the health of your mind, your body and your ability to sleep.

Losing just a few precious hours of sleep can affect your metabolism dramatically and can lead to weight gain. The increased weight can then make it harder for you to get good and restorative sleep at night and another vicious cycle is kicked off. Exercise is just one of the ways to help not only prevent the weight gain but to help get back on a better and more effective sleep cycle. The benefits of exercise on sleep include:

Giving you an outlet for some of your stress and frustrations.

Giving you enough movement to allow your body to feel "tired".

Allowing your muscles to stretch can actually help them to feel more pliable and more relaxed which can increase your comfort level.

Exercise can also put you more in tune with your body's signals. Once you can listen to these signals you should be able to recreate the exact balance you need for better sleep, more relaxed thoughts and a calmer approach to your entire life.

Unfortunately, when some people hear the word "exercise" they envision long distances of grueling runs, endlessly lifting heavy weights in a dark and sweaty gym or doing impossible to learn cardio routines to the sound of electro music. If any of that sounds good to you, have at it! If it sounds wretched and miserable, then take heart because there are other options. In fact, if you are new to exercise or are severely out of shape none of these are even right for you. (Once again, please remember that you should consult with your doctor before starting any exercise program). Lighter exercise programs are the best bet for the beginner not only because they are easier to manage but also because they will not cause injury and frustration. There are plenty of options to choose from so you should never have an exercise program that is boring or that you really do not like.

Walking is a perfect example of the nearly perfect exercise routine. It is something that nearly everybody can do at whatever level they are currently at. You control the speed and the distance. If you walk outside, you get the added advantage of getting fresh air, the chance to talk to some neighbors and maybe meet some new people and to really clear your head. Set a clear but achievable goal for yourself and off you go. You might say "I will walk around the block" or maybe just to the end of the road and back. Once that is too comfortable for you, you can increase the distance or increase the speed slightly. You might eventually work up to a jog. You might never get to that point. Either way, it is all right. You are doing something for yourself and your body and mind will appreciate it.

The advantages of walking are: no equipment to buy, can be done anywhere and can be done either alone or in groups. All that you need are a pair of supportive shoes. When the weather is bad you can walk on a treadmill or even in the local mall. When the weather is lovely you can walk outdoors. You can change your route every night or every few nights. You can take your kids, your spouse or just your pet or you can go alone, whatever feels best for you. In some cultures, a walk after the final meal of the night is traditional as it aids digestion. You can bring this to your own life- after you finish eating, load the dishwasher and then go off for your walk.

If walking is difficult for you, another option is swimming. Even floating in water is a relaxing experience. Researchers, desperately trying to unlock the stories behind the theta waves (See Chapter One), finally stumbled on the one waking experience that created them- floating in water. Even floating in a bathtub may be enough to create these very slow oscillating rhythms (theta waves are about 4-7 Hz). These waves are the most difficult to study because usually just as someone hits this particular rhythm they fall into a deeper sleep or they wake back up. Theta waves usually come in the period between drowsy/deeply relaxed and sleep and then again during sleep and waking up. These waves are associated with creative insight. If you have ever started to fall asleep when a sudden thought has overwhelmed you, you were experiencing theta waves. These are the same rhythms that inspire creative types like writers and artists. Even people who cannot swim at all can float-making it beyond perfect as an exercise.

You do not have to get sweaty and sore for something to count as exercise. You do not have to grunt and groan and pick up heavy things. Just do something active that makes you happy, moves your body and that you can continue to do every day. Just ten minutes of an exercise you love is better for you than nothing at all and may be more effective than an exercise that does not appeal to you.

Once it becomes a part of your routine you will realize how much you look forward to it if you cannot exercise for a day. If you find yourself coming up with excuses once again it might be time to find a new exercise to do. Keeping it fresh will keep your body and your mind improving all of the time and also keeps you from being bored.

Exercise increases your metabolism so keep that in mind when you plan your routine. Right after dinner is a great time but if you find that this interferes with sleep try to exercise earlier. Everyone is different, so find what works for you.

Chapter 11: Different Types Of Sleep Disorders, And What They Mean

Many people are embarrassed to see a doctor, or explain to work colleagues that they have sleep disorders. For something that is so common, it's surprising to note the lengths people will go to hide their personal   issues.

Think about it. If you had a child who was struggling with a sleep disorder, how much of that would you attribute to bad behavior? Would you be compassionate about it? It's the same with adults who feel it should be their duty to at least stay up later in the evening and answer emails or be readily available at all hours of the day.

People seem to check off brownie points when they are able to respond quickly after office hours, but it must be noted that this can lead to burnout.

Here is a list of conditions that are widely recognized, but not always discussed between friends and family.
Sleep   Apnea
Sleep Apnea is a disorder in which breathing repeatedly stops and starts, or periods of shallow breathing which occur more often than normal. They can last up to a few minutes, followed by loud choking sounds, snoring or other disruptive noises. In children, it may cause problems at school due to hyperactivity. It can also cause complications such as heart attacks, strokes and heart failures. The usual age of onset is between 55 and 60 years old. Sleep Apnea either occurs as obstructive Apnea, in which breathing is interrupted by a blockage in the air flow, or central sleep Apnea, in which regular unconscious

breath simply comes to a halt. The most common form is the former, and the risk factors include having a family history with the disorder. There are also factors such as having larger tonsils that may cause this. Some people are unaware they even have this condition, only to be told by family members that they disrupted other people's sleep in the night.

Insomnia

People with insomnia struggle with sleep, and their difficulties don't follow a consistent pattern. Sometimes they have problems falling asleep altogether, whereas on other nights, they may struggle to stay asleep once they've nodded off. They may wake up in the early hours, feeling neither well-rested nor alert. In turn, this affects the rest of their day, and as the hours go on, they feel tired and unable to do most physical or mental tasks.

They can feel incredibly lethargic, and people with insomnia may even become irritable and have moods swings. Insomnia can cause anxiety and can also lead to schizophrenia, chronic depression, and other disorders. If a person's work performance or daily functioning begins to slip, insomnia may be the source. But what is the cause of insomnia? It can result from many different factors, and it may even be a short-term stress related condition. Most often, insomnia is an indicator of an underlying and untreated condition.

Imagine that your child or sibling has a health condition; falling asleep could mean missing vital changes in their well-being. Other factors can include sleeping in a room that is too loud, or in the wrong type of bed or mattress that is too firm, too soft, too high, etc.

Another important element may be that you're not getting enough exercise, so if your job suddenly requires driving, where before it required walking, your sleep rhythm and routine can be thrown out of sync. Other risks include abusing drugs or alcohol, especially high-alert substances such as cocaine, or MDMA. One psychological cause may be having nightmares because of a previous trauma. These recurring dreams should be treated as soon as possible. Especially frustrating is when you pay $60 for an hour's session, only to receive the same advice you would get from a $7 book!

Other factors may be chronic pain that a person learns to live with during the day, but the ache becomes distracting at night, especially when they are alone in the dark. Women who experience menopause and have hormonal changes can also suffer from interrupted bouts of sleep. Insomnia can be a sign of Alzheimer's disease, because early symptoms often indicate disruption to the brain. Research also shows that insomnia can be caused by too much 'screen time', or using electronic devices before bed. This can be especially problematic for younger generations.

They may stay awake messaging friends without regulating the amount of time they spend online.

After all, teenagers can be rebellious and hide their phones or tablets in or around their bed.

Taking anti-depressants too early (or too late) in the day can cause stages of insomnia. This can also lead to poor concentration at school or work, a lack of coordinated body movement or other accidents.

Insomnia can be transient or chronic;

primary insomnia is a standalone problem, whereas secondary insomnia can point to a different condition. It can also be classified by how severely it affects the individual, and what impact it has on their sleep cycle. So really, treating it is only part of the wider issue: another problem is identifying what type of insomnia the person has. Some well researched reports reveal that using blackout blinds, sleeping away from an easily reachable phone, bathing before bed and establishing some resemblance of a night-time routine helps a great deal.

Narcolepsy

This is a chronic sleep disorder which is characterized by sudden, overwhelming drowsiness and attacks of sleep. People with this condition find it very difficult to stay awake, regardless of what they're doing. It can cause very serious disruptions to daily routines.

People may fall asleep without warning, anywhere, even while in mid-conversation. Eventually, even after you've woken up feeling refreshed, you begin to feel tired again. You may also experience decreased alertness, and drowsiness throughout the day. It's hard to focus, and it makes it very difficult for anyone to concentrate. There can also be a sudden loss of muscle tone that accompanies it, which may even result in slurred speech and weaker muscles.

It is an uncontrollable condition, and some people experience this side-effect much worse than others, having some episodes occur daily when they laugh or feel extreme emotion.

Hypersomnia

Then there is hypersomnia, which refers to excessive time spent sleeping, or increased amounts of sleepiness during the day. This is a similar condition in which a person finds it hard to stay awake. This could be a result of not getting a good night's rest, being overweight, drug abuse, alcohol or a result of a head injury. Some studies have shown that genetics play a key role in developing hypersomnia, with tranquilizer drugs making the condition worse.

Jet **Lag**
This is also known as the 'time zone change' syndrome or desynchronosis. It occurs mainly when people travel frequently across time-zones, or when their sleep is disrupted due to work shifts. It is also a circadian rhythm disorder, which happens when there is a disruption to the body clock. Symptoms are more severe when travelling to the East, compared with travelling to the West. Jet lag can be the leading cause of

insomnia, irritability, and headaches while flying. It also affects children less than it affects adults.

Restless Leg Syndrome
This disorder, also known by its abbreviated term (RLS), is the overwhelming need for leg movement, especially when someone is lying down or very still. As you can imagine (or maybe you already know first-hand), Restless Leg Syndrome seriously effects sleep patterns. It is unclear what the root cause is, but the lack of iron deficiency and dopamine contribute to constant leg movement which results in a lack of sleep and much needed rest for the body. Some prescribed medications can cause dizzy spells, but natural remedies such as yoga and dopamine increasing supplements may be more beneficial. A focus on gut health may also be helpful. If you have RLS, you probably know the

following symptoms all too well. When you're in bed, you feel an urge or even a sharp sensation, which stings and forces you to move your legs. When you do get out of bed to pace up and down, the relief does not last, and it's not long before you have to move again. It actually affects ten percent of the American population. Perhaps a better method for this neurological sensory disorder is to try supplements and natural remedies. Supplements and remedies may temporarily stop the pain, but it should make it easier for individuals to get some sleep at night.

Chapter 12: Treating Sleep Apnea

Sleep apnea can be treated. There are different approaches for the treatment of this disorder. You can start by managing it at home.

Home Treatment for Sleep Apnea

There are two ways on how you can manage sleep apnea at home and these are through changing your lifestyle and by changing your sleeping habits as well. Try these simple changes:

· Lifestyle Change

o Weight Loss – One of the risk factors of sleep apnea is being overweight. If you have this disorder and have sleep apnea, then losing weight may help. Studies showed that losing weight decreases the number of times that you stop breathing during your sleep.

o   Reduce alcohol and some medications that can worsen the symptoms of sleep apnea. Sedatives are the one of the types of medications that may worsen sleep apnea symptoms.

o   Get enough sleep. Sleep apnea may be more observable in those people with lack of sleep.

o   Stop smoking. It is the nicotine that is found in smoke that causes the muscles in the airways to relax. Stopping smoking will help make the muscles function well.

o   Treat problems that cause difficulty of breathing such as stuffy nose.

Lifestyle changes may help manage sleep apnea. However, if this does not solve the problem, then you can also do it with the following changes in your sleeping habits:

· Sleeping Habits Changes

o Sleep on your side. Sleeping on your side will help in managing mild sleep apnea.

o Raise your head while sleeping. Try placing a cervical pillow. This will help in holding your head in an elevated position.

With the changes in lifestyle and sleeping habits, you may be able to manage mild sleep apnea. However, if sleep apnea persists, there are other options that you can discuss with your health care provider so that your sleep apnea can be managed and its complications prevented.

· Therapies

Here are some of the options that your doctor may advice you to have.

Continuous Positive Airway Pressure (CPAP)

This is one way of treating moderate to severe sleep apnea. This is done with the use of a device that will assist you in breathing while you are sleeping. This device is designed to give you compressed air through a mask. The compressed air will prevent closing of the throat. This has been found to be an effective non-surgical choice of treatment for people with sleep apnea.

CPAP may be uncomfortable at the start, but through time, you may just learn to adjust to the mask that you will be required to wear. You can also talk to your physician on how long you will be undergoing the treatment or you may change the mask into something that you are more comfortable with.

There are disadvantages in using CPAP as well. The first week of using it may be uncomfortable yet it is easy enough to get used to it. Some of the other disadvantages are as follows:

o Dry nose

o Irritated eyes

o Sore throat

o Abdominal bloating

o Nasal congestion

These risks are manageable with the adjustments done to improve CPAP therapy. You can use humidifiers to avoid dryness of throat and nose, or use nasal decongestants to avoid nasal congestion. You just have to speak with your physician about CPAP to make it more comfortable to use.

Adjustable Airway Pressure Devices

If you are uncomfortable with CPAP then there are other choices for you. There are other devices that can help you with sleep apnea. This device makes use of another airway pressure that adjusts while you are sleeping. There are devices that deliver bi-level positive airway pressure (BPAP) that provides different pressures when you inhale or exhale.

Expiratory Positive Airway Pressure

This device is available in single use units. It is placed on each nostril before you go to sleep. The device allows you to inhale freely but during exhalation, the air passes through small holes that leave pressure on the airway to keep it open. This device is a good replacement for CPAP as it reduces snoring and improves on daytime sleepiness.

Adaptive Servo-Ventilation

This also makes use of a device that will send signals on how it would regulate airflow so that it prevents apnea while you sleep.

Dental Devices

There are dental devices that are used to treat sleep apnea. Devices such as a tongue retaining device and a mandibular retaining device will help in opening your airway. This is done by a dentist and you should have it fitted to avoid feeling any discomfort while using it.

Treating Underlying Medical Condition

In cases of sleep apnea that may be caused by an underlying medical condition especially those that involve neuromuscular or heart disorders, prior treatment of these diseases should first be done. If sleep apnea improves with the treatment of these diseases, then no other treatment specifically for sleep apnea is necessary.

Supplemental Oxygen

Having supplemental oxygen while you sleep will help you deal with sleep apnea. You have choices on how supplemental oxygen can be delivered to your lungs.

These are just therapies that may help you manage sleep apnea if changes in lifestyle and sleeping habits do not seem to be working out. You can also combine these therapies with the changes that you are doing for better results. However, if still sleep apnea is unmanageable despite your efforts to change and use these devices, then invasive procedures may be necessary. This is the last option when all the other treatments failed.

· Surgery

In cases of obstructive sleep apnea, surgery may be required. Here are some of the surgeries that you may undergo depending on the case of obstructive sleep apnea that you have.

Uvulopalatopharyngoplasty (UPPP)

This procedure is done to enlarge the airway in the retro palatal area. This is done by excising a part of the uvula in the posterior aspect of the soft palate and the lateral pharyngeal wall mucosa. This procedure is done together with adenotonsillectomy and/or resection of the tongue to enlarge the airway. This has shown to be 40-50% effective. However, this may fail if other airways are not given attention to. This should be done only by experienced surgeons as this may have unwanted results when not done properly. Dysphagia, velopharyngeal insufficiency, hyper nasal speech, residual obstructive sleep apnea, and nasopharyngeal stenosis may result from the said surgery. There are modifications done with this kind of surgery to minimize post-operative complications.

Uvuloplasty with Laser Assistance

This procedure is done to treat snoring and has been reported to have 80-85% success rate. This is an outpatient procedure done under local anesthesia with decreased post-operative complications brought about by the invasive procedure. However, in a recent study, the effectiveness showed that only 27% had good response while 34% had poor response and the other 30% got worse after the surgery. Thus, it is very important to discuss the procedure with an expert. You may also undergo a series of imaging tests to determine the right procedure for you.

Uvulopalatal Flap

This is done to widen the oropharyngeal airway by retracting the uvula to the junction of the soft and the hard palate. This procedure is contraindicated if the palate or the uvula is bulky as this procedure may just create more obstruction. This is more preferred compared to UPPP as this has lesser post-operative pain because of the lesser stitches that UPPP and the laser therapy has.

Nasal Reconstruction

This is done to patients whose obstructive sleep apnea is caused solely by nasal obstruction. This surgery would be very effective. This is done to patients who have an airway obstruction brought about by its anatomy. Septoplasty, septorhinoplasty, cryotherapy and laser vaporization are just some of the procedures under nasal reconstruction.

Adenotonsillectomy

This is done in children to control or manage loud snoring and restlessness during night time sleep. Palatal surgery may even be done on children who are severely obese.

Palatal Surgery

This is a surgery wherein many of the oropharyngeal structures are involved. This involves the tonsils, the tonsillar pillars, the uvula and the posterior tonsillar pillars. This may involve excision or removal of certain parts to widen the airway.

Implants

Implants are placed in the soft palate in the form of plastic rods. This is done under local anesthesia. This is an option procedure for those people with mild sleep apnea that cannot tolerate CPAP.

Dental Devices

If a person with sleep apnea cannot tolerate CPAP then dental devices may be given. Here are the dental implants that can help people with sleep apnea.

o Mandibular Adjustment Device (MAD) – this is a device that looks like a sports mouth guard. It forces the lower jaw forward and slightly downward to keep the airway open. This is widely used to treat sleep apnea.

o Tongue Retraining Device (RTD) – this is like a splint for the tongue to keep the airway open.

There are certain benefits that dental devices have. These have been shown to lessen apneas in patients. They work best when the person lies on his back. It improves sleep and reduces snoring or its loudness in some patients.

Tracheostomy

For people who have life threatening sleep apnea, an alternative airway should be made and this is done through tracheostomy. This is a procedure wherein a surgeon will be inserting a tube through an incision made in your neck. This will become your temporary airway.

· Medications

There are also medications that are being administered for people with sleep apnea. Such drugs are given not to treat sleep apnea but to manage the accompanying symptoms and disorders. Medications include:

o Modafinil – this is a medication of choice approved by the FDA for narcolepsy and is also given to people with extreme sleepiness caused by sleep apnea. However, this should be used in conjunction with other sleep apnea treatment such as CPAP.

o Thyroid hormones are also given to those people with sleep apnea and low thyroid hormones.

o Intranasal corticosteroids – may be helpful in children with sleep apnea.

Chapter 13: Sleep Meditations

If you have been through one of those sleepless nights, you'll definitely agree that putting the mind at rest in order to fall asleep is more difficult to do than what you may have originally thought. The second chapter of this book taught you some mind and body relaxation techniques. However, attaining a relaxed mind and body is just the start of getting the quality and quantity of sleep that is labeled as ideal. Our ability to control thoughts at will plays a more significant role in the attainment of such a goal.

Meditation is one of the best ways around the dilemma being mentioned above. You'll discover that as the night goes deeper and you are still awake, frustration levels increase and anxiety sets in. This is what disturbs the flow of thoughts that you have. As you can see, thought processes that have been slowed down through conscious efforts would pave the way to the initiation of a truly restful sleep.

The effectiveness of meditation in helping us sleep and overcome insomnia would depend on many factors. One is about the amount of practice that you are willing to do. Most of the time, you have to practice meditation techniques many times throughout the day before you can get any good progress during the night. Sleeping pattern is another factor here. There are people who are used to staying up 4 hours or more before feeling relaxed and ready to sleep. Some are able to fall asleep just after a few minutes of lying down in bed.

The biggest factor here, however, is the kind of meditation that would be chosen.

There are different types of meditation that you could choose from. The types that promote mental alertness should be avoided. Such meditation types include those that are taught in yoga, Zen, and tai-chi. By doing these meditation types 15 minutes before going to bed; you will reduce your chances of immediately falling asleep.

The most recommended type is under the broad category called as "mindful-meditation". It basically slows down the flow of thoughts coming into your mind. It also gives you the power to put the pace of your thoughts on the right track in case it wanders off. We all have this thing called as "inner chatter" in our minds and if this can be controlled (slowed down or calmed down); we can achieve that greater level of relaxation. After this, you can proceed to specific types of meditation that could match your actual needs.

Under the "mindful-meditation" category, three very effective techniques could be used for the attainment of high quality sleep. You can try out any of the following:

Mindful Breathing Technique–The process is quite easy as you will just pay attention to the pattern of your natural breathing. By doing this, you actually take your mind off thoughts that could disrupt the process of falling asleep. This is most effective if used together with music and guided visual imagery.

Body Scan Technique – This is very similar to the PMR (Progressive Muscle Relaxation) method mentioned on the 2nd chapter of this book. Start out by using technique #1 and then turn your attention to your toes. Visualize and feel it getting heavy and sinking into the bed. Move up and do the whole process all over again on your lower leg. Proceed upwards until you have "scanned" all of your body.

Combination Style Technique: As the name suggests, you can choose parts of different meditation and relaxation techniques here. Just remember to avoid those that add up to the alertness level of your mind and body. You can refer to chapter 2 of this book for a complete list of those techniques that can be combined.

Before you try any of the techniques mentioned above, it is necessary that you set realistic expectations about the results that can be obtained. If you haven't tried meditation yet, practice it. The help of a professional sleep therapist will definitely help, but it is not a requirement.

Chapter 14: Change Your Diet

The sleep disorders stated in the book, most notably insomnia can't be cured only through efficient time management, exercise and stress control. One of the causes of these stress disorders is poor diet. Poor diet means that the body is not getting enough vitamins, minerals and carbohydrates to function properly. Here are some food items that should become your main focus after reading this chapter.

- **Honey**: This is one of nature's most valuable gift to us. Honey is known to alleviate stress and induce sleep in the body as it contains specifics amino acids that trigger such a hormonal response. The hormones, i.e. serotonin and melatonin cause a person to feel good about himself which in turn lead to a calmer sleeping pattern. Honey is not the only source of this amino acid, but it is by far the most widely available one so try to consume a tablespoon of honey just before you go to bed, 2 days a week.

- **Legumes & Green Vegetables:** While honey does a great job at injecting tranquility, legumes and fresh vegetables can have a serene effect on nerves in the muscles. This leads to a natural drowsy feeling and thus a good night's sleep. The main reason behind this is the magnesium content in green vegetables which is an excellent nutrient for the muscles. Therefore, you should try to make magnesium rich food items a part of your diet like wheat bran, almonds, seeds & legumes, whole grain, etc. Try to keep it as natural as possible and stay away from processed foods.

-   **Milk:** Many of you might already be using this remedy in your quest to sleep. Milk has long been considered a viable source of triggering sleep. Children who are given milk right before bed find it much easier to sleep. Chemicals in milk can increase the level of serotonin in the body and thus work in the same way as honey. Calcium is one of key minerals here, so you're not just limited to milk but you can shift to other dairy products as well. For lactose intolerant individuals, including cereal, tofu and salmon can be a good idea.

-   **Oats:** Oats are a complete meal. They are highly nutritious, rich in fiber and wonderful stimulants. They can replenish the body's energy supply with smoothness and without any side effects. One of their many benefits is making sleep deprived individuals feel calm & serene. Oats don't work overnight and require time to kick in so don't start expecting any miracles.

-   **Bananas:** Bananas aren't known for prompting sleep. Instead, they contain Vitamin B6 that can keep you from waking up randomly at night. You can consume bananas either raw or in the form of some dessert. A simple recipe is as follows: blend 1 – 2 bananas with a cup of normal/soy milk & add some ice to it. Other food items with similar effects include bell peppers, tuna, spinach and chicken.

-   **Almonds:** These are one of the top natural remedies to treating insomnia. Almonds are a great source of proteins that can regulate blood sugar and ensure deeper sleep cycles. One tablespoon of almond butter added in any dish or eaten raw would be enough to regulate your sleep.

- **Premature soybeans:** Are you one of those people who enjoy a salty snack before going to bed? Well, I have for you a snack that will not only satisfy your cravings but will also help your sleep. Soybeans are estrogen-like food items that can bring down the intensity with which nighttime flashes hit you. These flashes are one of the main reasons a person wakes up for no reason at nights. Grab two cups of shelled soybeans, toss them into a blender or a food processor along with a few drops of olive oil and blend until a smooth mixture forms; enjoy.

In addition to adding all these things to your diet, there are also a few that you should readily phase out.

- **Caffeine:** People who drink too much coffee or tea will find it difficult at times to fall asleep at a regular time. The situation is much worse for someone who consumes caffeine containing drinks right before going to bed. This will keep him up till late night, which will ultimately lead to shorter sleep duration. Caffeine has such an effect because it blocks out adenosine, a neurotransmitter that promotes sleep.

People who suffer from insomnia should try to avoid caffeine as much as possible as the effects can go on for hours. A gradual approach to caffeine elimination will be much more fruitful compared to going cold turkey as caffeine withdrawal leads to irritation, headache and fatigue.

-    **Smoking:** Nicotine is a major constituent of cigarettes. It is also a central nervous system stimulant and this means only one thing; it can cause insomnia. Nicotine is known to raise one's heart rate, blood pressure and trigger fast brain wave activity that causes wakefulness. If you can't get rid of this bad habit altogether, at least don't smoke 1 – 2 hours before going to bed.

- **Alcohol:** This is one of the most loved but at the same time most hated drink on the planet. Alcohol depresses the nervous system at least for a few hours. Not just that, it can suppress REM sleep and trigger frequent awakenings at night. Drinkers have also complained of frightening dreams while 10% of chronic insomnia cases are linked to alcohol abuse.

Drinking at night can increase the chances of drowsiness during other parts of the day. Even a single drink can make a sleep-deprived person loss control. In an automobile, this can turn into a fatal combo.

Chapter 15: Environment And Sleep

Changing Your Environment

If you are genuinely interested in increasing your quality of sleep, then it is highly recommended that you alter your environment for the better. Your environment refers to you social interactions, as well the environmental triggers that affect your mental, physical and emotional state, and ultimately, your sleep cycle. This chapter will review the following sections: Physical environment, sound, lighting, electronics, social interaction.

Physical Environment

The comfort of your bed and pillow affect the quality of your sleep, as well as your capacity to fall asleep. It is also important that you set your home to the proper temperature in order to prevent restlessness. Try to sleep in comfortable clothes, and choose bedding that is compatible with your skin.

Attempt to make you physical environment as comfortable and as aesthetically appealing as possible in order to facilitate sleep and increase the duration and quality of sleep.

Sound and Lighting

Improper sound and lighting can induce states of sleeplessness. For example, when you are exposed to noise levels that are between 40-70 decibels, you impair your capacity to fall asleep. However, if you have long been exposed to a sound, such as traffic sounds, while asleep, eliminating these sounds can disrupt sleep as well.

Light is one of the most critical factors in our sleep cycles, and it helps regulate circadian rhythms. Hence, before sleeping, try to eliminate bright lighting. It is critical that during the day, you undergo significant bright light exposure. But during sleep, you must expose yourself to sufficient darkness and eliminate as much light as possible.

Electronics

Electronics are seamlessly integrated into the fabric of our daily life. Not to mention, they can affect your sleep cycles. Some of your favorite devices can even deprive you of a quality night of sleep. Because electronic devices project bright light, they hinder the brain's ability to fall asleep. So, if you want to sleep, do not use these devices shortly before bed.

Social Interactions

It is no secret that your interaction with others can affect your quality of sleep, as well as your ability to fall asleep. If you experience rage, an argument, shock, severe anxiety, or serious emotional turmoil within hours of falling asleep, you will experience restlessness and sleeplessness. Here are a few situations that may disrupt a normal sleep cycle:

• An argument with a coworker or significant other can spark high levels of physiological arousal, including elevated heart rate, blood pressure, and respiration.

• A serious disappointment can make you ruminate and engage in repetitive thought patterns that disrupt sleep.

• Intense emotional distress can disrupt sleep for obvious reasons,

Many of these emotional states derive from interactions with others. So, for the sake of having a healthy night's sleep, try to engage in the following behaviors:

• Engage in conflict resolution to decrease conflict. High levels of negative emotional arousal disrupt sleep cycles. The negative effects of an argument can linger for hours, assuming control of your emotional state and your thought patterns, as well. Furthermore, it can impair your ability to relax.

• Focus on positive interactions and foster healthy relationships that do not disrupt bodily functions. Positive interactions have a healing and calming effect on the mind. And the more relaxed your physical and mental state is, the easier it will be to fall asleep.

• Develop healthy coping mechanisms for life's disappointment. By doing so, will will be able to emotionally regulate and reduce the emotional effects associated with certain situations. This will enable you to assume control of your emotional state and relax before bed.

As you can see, what you expose yourself to in the outside world is just as important as the physical mechanisms inside your body. Sleep requires an internal and external effort that maximizes your environmental surroundings and sleep patterns.

Chapter 16: The Science Of Falling Asleep

Sleep is a natural part of life, but do you know how and why it occurs? Many questions about sleep have been answered in the name of science, but there are certain aspects of it that are still a mystery. However, let us discuss the parts that you must know, especially if falling sleep has already become a nightly struggle.

The Different Stages of Sleep

Neuroscientists, such as those at the Washington University in St. Louis, categorize the process of falling sleep and sleep per se into five stages: pre-sleep, transitional sleep (or stage 1), non-REM sleep (or stage 2), slow wave sleep (or stages 3 and 4), and REM sleep. Each stage is discussed briefly and in a not-too-technical way below:

The Pre-Sleep Stage. This stage is where your"bedtime routine"transpires. Specifically, it is the time when you are just about to get ready for sleep. You turn off the lights, get comfortable in your bed and close your eyes.

As you wait for sleep to occur, your brain enters a transitional period called"quiet wakefulness."In other words, it softly shifts between thoughts regarding the outside world and your inner mind, with the latter progressively becoming more dominant. These inner thoughts consist of either self-reflection or works of pure imagination, or both.

Eventually, or approximately after 7 minutes, the mind moves on to the Transitional Sleep Stage.

The Transitional Sleep Stage. When you start to daydream with less effort, you are most likely in Stage 1 or the transitional sleep stage. It is a curious state to be in, because you sometimes experience what are called"hypnogogic hallucinations"in the form of unusual yet vivid mental images and sensations. It is unknown how long the transitional sleep stage lasts, but some guess it is between 5 and 10 minutes. If uninterrupted, you can then proceed to the non-REM Sleep stage.

The non-REM Sleep Stage. This stage, which is also referred to as Stage 2, is when your body temperature drops and your heart rates becomes slower. This also reduces your brain's ability to perceive your external environment. For instance, the music you may have been listening to while in bed progressively fades away at this point.

REM stands for"rapid eye movement,"which happens when you are dreaming. In this case, you are not in dreamland yet. This stage lasts for approximately 20 minutes before you move on to the next stage.

The Slow Wave Sleep Stage. When people are talking about a long, dreamless sleep, they may be referring to this stage, formerly categorized as Stages 3 and 4. Also called"deep sleep," it is when your brain emits Delta Waves, or deep, slow brain waves. It lasts for roughly half an hour before finally moving on to REM sleep.

The REM Sleep Stage. As you continue to go deeper into your sleep cycle, your mind rewards you by allowing you to enter the dream world. During this stage, your voluntary muscles are relaxed to the point of immobility, so that you will not"act out"your dreams. Your brain, on the other hand, becomes more active. In your first complete sleep cycle, this stage will last for approximately 10 minutes. However, the more consecutive sleep cycles you have, the longer each REM sleep stage becomes.

The stages between transitional sleep and REM sleep last for approximately 1 hour and 30 minutes. This is known as one"sleep cycle."Throughout the night, you go through the cycle repeatedly until you wake up naturally or you are jolted from it (as in the case of those who use an alarm clock).

How to Determine the Number of Hours You Need to Sleep

The number of hours you need to sleep is largely determined by the number of cycles your mind and body needs. Keep in mind that yours may be different from the others.

For instance, some can get by with only three uninterrupted sleep cycles (or 4 hours and 30 minutes of sleep) each night, while others need at least five (or 7 hours and 30 minutes).

To find out how many hours or sleep cycles you need, take note of the approximate time you fell asleep the previous night and the time you naturally woke up the following morning. Do this for several nights (ideally for a week). By the end of this experiment, you can gauge the number of hours you need to set aside for sleep every night. If you cannot afford to not use an alarm clock in the morning, you can do this experiment on the weekends when you can allow yourself to wake up naturally.

After determining the number of hours you need, use it as the foundation to create a bedtime routine. For example, if you noticed that you usually fall asleep at around 11 p.m. and then naturally wake up at around 6:30 a.m., then that means your body needs 7 hours and 30 minutes of sleep, or five sleep cycles.

If you have to be up by 5 a.m. for work, however, this means you need to count back and set your bedtime earlier. In this case, that will be on or before 9:30 p.m.

Aside from this, you should also factor in the number of minutes it takes for you to fall asleep. For instance, if you realized that you fall asleep 20 minutes after getting to bed, then make sure to set aside this amount of time to be in bed.

Hopefully a lot of the questions on sleep in your mind have been answered now that you have a clearer picture of how it naturally works. Use this knowledge to establish habits that will help you fall into it effortlessly. If you do not know where to begin, then do not worry for the succeeding chapters in this book will help you each step of the way.

Chapter 17: Basics Of Sleep Apnea And Snoring

Sleep apnea is a chronic, potentially serious disorder where your sleep is disrupted by breathing pauses or when you experience shallow breathing during sleep. Breathing pauses can occur for a few seconds to several minutes, with a frequency of around 30 times or more in one hour. When you pause breathing, the level of oxygen delivered to the brain is below normal. The brain then responds to this by disrupting your sleep so you jumpstart your breathing. A loud choking or gasping sound accompanies this. Often times, this causes you to move out of deep sleep into a lighter sleep, or you may be awakened.

What are the types of sleep apnea?

Obstructive sleep apnea is the most common type. Snoring ensues because the soft tissues at the back of the throat relax during sleep and block the airway. Moreover, allergies or other medical conditions that result to nasal congestion and blockage may contribute to obstructive sleep apnea. In this condition, you may not be aware of your awakenings.

Central sleep apnea involves the central nervous system and is not as common as obstructive sleep apnea. It occurs when the brain fails to activate the muscles that control your breathing. People with this condition seldom snore and are often aware of their sleep being disrupted by apnea.

Complex sleep apnea is obstructive sleep apnea and central sleep apnea combined.

Who can have sleep apnea?

Sleep apnea can affect male, female, the young or the old. However, there are particular risk factors associated with each type.

You are at risk for obstructive sleep apnea if you are:

65 years old or above

Male

Overweight

Smoker

Has a family member suffering from sleep apnea

Hispanic, Pacific Islander, or Black

Other factors may include the following physical attributes:

Thick neck

Enlarged tonsils or adenoids (common in children)

Deviated septum

Receding chin

You are at risk for central sleep apnea if you are:

65 years old or above

suffering from a serious medical condition (such as stroke, heart disease, neurological problems, or brainstem or spinal injury)

What are the signs and symptoms?

Sleep apnea may root from a serious disorder; therefore, it is necessary to consult your doctor. However, sleep apnea is often undiagnosed because the prominent symptoms can manifest while you are sleeping. You may need the help of a sleep partner to observe your sleeping habits. You may also set up an audio or video recording of yourself during sleep. Snoring may indicate sleep apnea, as well as the following:

While asleep

shallow breathing

breathing pauses

gasping for air or choking

awakenings, feeling confused

At daytime

Dry mouth or sore throat upon waking up

Morning headaches

Extreme sleepiness

Feeling of poor sleep quality

Poor concentration, attention or memory

Mood swings

Recent weight gain

Is it sleep apnea or just snoring?

Snoring may indicate sleep apnea, but not all those who have sleep apnea snore. Furthermore, snoring does not automatically mean one has sleep apnea. The major difference lies on the fact that snoring does not likely affect the quality of sleep, thus, daytime symptoms may not be present.

What are the causes of snoring?

The way you snore indicates the cause of snoring. By correctly determining how you snore, you are closer to knowing the appropriate cure for your condition.

Snoring while the mouth is closed indicate tongue problem

Snoring while the mouth is open may be linked to tissues at the back of your throat.

Snoring while sleeping on your back is a milder problem and may indicate the need for a change in positioning, improvement in sleep habits and lifestyle changes

Snoring in all sleep positions is more severe and may necessitate a more comprehensive management.

What can treat sleep apnea and snoring?

The objective of treating sleep apnea is to be able to re-establish a regular breathing pattern during sleep and to alleviate symptoms such as snoring and symptoms of poor sleep quality. Obstructive sleep apnea and snoring can be treated by making changes in your bedtime habits and lifestyle, as well as performing throat exercises. Clinical treatments may also be considered, which may include the use of dental appliance, breathing devices and even surgery. Medications are only used to treat daytime sleepiness associated with sleep apnea, but does not cure the apnea itself In cases of central apnea, treating the underlying medical condition, such as neuromuscular or heart disorder, is necessary.

Chapter 18: Self-Help Therapy

Other sleeping disorders may require the help of a medical professional, but you can still improve your sleeping habit on your own.

Keep a Sleep Diary

Keeping a sleep diary can greatly help you identify the symptoms of your sleeping disorder. It can also help you pinpoint the habits that affect your sleep. Your sleep diary should contain the following:

o Time of your sleep and when you wake up

o Total time of sleep

o Mood before going to bed

o Time you spent awake

o Any medication you took along with the dosage

Putting as much detail on your sleep diary can reveal how your behavior affects your sleep. Observe your sleeping pattern very well over a period of time.

Improve Sleep Habits

A good sleeping routine can drastically improve your sleeping habits and can help you attain a better quality of sleep. Try to sleep during the same time every day even on weekends. Make sleep a top priority. People often neglect sleep whenever they encounter stressful situations.

Turn off your phone, computer and TV few hours before sleeping. This will prevent any light from disturbing your sleep.

Make sure that you are warm enough. The ideal temperature for sleeping is 65 degrees.

Take a warm soothing bath before you sleep. Warm water can relax your muscles. Use relaxing scents. Vanilla, lavender and chamomile scents are very relaxing and can also help reduce stress.

Relaxing music can also help some people sleep, but make sure to set the timer in your music player so that it doesn't play all night.

Create an environment for sleeping

Sleeping can be difficult if your room is not conducive for relaxation. Here are some tips in making your bedroom a suitable place for sleep.

Location. Place your bed in a quieter spot. It is also important to use your bed strictly for sleeping and sex only. This will condition your body to interpret the bed as a place of relaxation.

Orderliness. A messy room can disrupt your sense of relaxation. Avoid any unnecessary clutter and make sure that you have enough storage space for your things. Remember that disorder and relaxation does not go together.

Color. Choose light and soft colors for your room. Green is a soothing color that reminds people of nature. Blue resembles relaxing atmosphere. Avoid loud colors. They are best kept for accessories and to make your room lively.

Light. Do not place your bed directly below your main light. A light that has shimmer in it is best. Lamps with crystals can remind you of stars while small candle lights can evoke memories of romantic dinners.

Materials. Try to surround yourself with comfortable materials like fluffy pillows and soft rugs.

Chapter 19: Importance Of Sleep

"Your life is a reflection of your sleep, and how you sleep is a reflection of your life" – Dr Rafael Pelayo, Senior Professor, Psychiatry and Behavioral Sciences, Stanford - Centre for Sleep Sciences and Medicines.

Sleep acts as a balm that massages our subconscious, soothing our innermost self. A person with good sleep at night is a person reborn the next morning.

Sleep is to good health and well-being as breathing is to our very existence. The amount of time spent in bed, watching the back of your eye lids is going to decide the nature of your time spent out of bed. The quality of your valuable lifetime and safety revolves around a nucleus called SLEEP.

During sleep, you may look limp, but your body works constantly to support healthy functioning of the brain and maintenance of your physical health. In children and adolescent sleep plays a critical role in supporting growth and development.

Sleep deficiency can result in abrupt consequences (sudden accidents or mishaps) or slow corrosion (sluggish and stagnant mental and motor skills). For example, persistent sleep deficiency increases your risk for some chronic health problems. It can adversely affect your thought patterns, working patterns, learning and retention, and interpersonal relations.

To maintain a firm equilibrium between body and mind, adequate amount of sleep is necessary varying according to different age group.

Babies (0-2 months old)
12-18 hours

Infants (3-11 months old)
14-15 Hours

Toddlers (1-3 years old)
12-14 Hours

Pre-School (3-5 years old)
11-13 Hours

School-Aged Children 5-10 years old)
10-11 Hours

Teens (11-17 years old)
8-9 Hours

Adults
7-9 Hours

Chronic Sleep Disorders may lead to a number of serious medical conditions, mental or physical. Studies have proved sleep to be of utmost priority as good sleeping habits leads to longevity in age and healthier lives in terms of handling stress or strengthening your immune system

Sleep is a basic human need which needs serious attention without which our life will be reduced to nothing but a bundle of anxieties, unproductivity and physical ill-health

David Beniof, a famous American novelist, Screen-writer and Television Producer has quoted: "I have always envied people who sleep easily. Their brains must be cleaner, the floorboards of the skull well swept, all the little monsters closed up in a steamer trunk at the foot of the bed"

Common Misconceptions

Even though about one third of our lives are spent on sleep, it is surprising that most people live with myths about sleep, not realizing that clearing the smoke can benefit them in innumerable ways. Here are some of the major misbeliefs that one must sort before searching for a delightful sleep experience.

Tiredness is synonymous to sleep

While the former may lead to the latter, the latter may has its reasons. Tiredness is a signal that the body or mind needs rest. Overexerting oneself may find one of the solutions in sleep but sleep also depends on many other factors like sleep clock, medications at times etc

Sleep breaks when eyes open

Physical indicators do not confirm that the body is completely conscious. It takes time to switch gears from a state of sleep to complete state of awakening. Do not jump to a conclusion that lack of immediate freshness after waking up means inadequate sleep

Backlog of sleep can be compensated for

In todays' hectic lifestyles and schedules, it is a struggle to cope up with sleep. You mostly fill the buffer on weekends. This way the short term deficit may get fulfilled but the problem lies in its long term impact. The body slowly collects these small deposits over a period of time showing signs of sluggishness physical, exhaustion, behavioral fluctuations etc

If not eight hours, our sleep is useless

It is an average number of hours that we must fulfil, but each individual has a different sleep clock depending on their life commitments. It is the quality of sleep along with about six to eight hours of resting that are important.

Snoring, a sign of prosperity

One of the greatest myths is that snoring indicates satisfactory sleep. It is not so. There is an undercurrent health hazard that goes along with it. If left undiagnosed it can lead to chronic respiratory and cardiac problems.

Sleep goes strictly by the 'day and night' norm

People condition their lives to the night and day clock. The reality is that sleep needs attention when your body demands it. Stress levels may scream into your subconscious for more sleep but you consciously ignore it considering that the time is not appropriate.

Hours of sleep directly proportional to quality of sleep

Forced sleep may bring you to fall back on your pillow but eyes shut are no guarantee to a fulfilling sleep. Factors like bad dreams, frequent interruptions in the form of call of nature or maybe alarms etc. may hinder the quality of sleep. You may wake up feeling dissatisfied even after a night long sleep

Caffeine induces sleep

You need to separate addiction from need. Those who propagate it as a sleep inducer have conditioned their need to it. The facts are far from this. Caffeine products are stimulants! They give an initial energy boost after which you suddenly feel drained. You may blame a stressful day for a sleepless night but it is the caffeine intake in the day that tells on us even at night.

Chapter 20: How Does Your Diet Affect Your Sleep?

We need to know what our body does to induce sleep before we examine what the best foods are for a successful sleep cycle. There are four main minerals that aid sleeping. Tryptophan, Magnesium, Calcium, and B6. It is possible to ingest these minerals in supplements, but the best way is to add them to your diet.

Here are the best foods to add to your diet for each of the main minerals

1)Tryptophan: This is an amino acid that encourages your pineal gland to produce melatonin. As your natural bedtime approaches your body will automatically release melatonin into your bloodstream and help you prepare for sleep.

- Organic meats: Lamb, beef, liver, chicken, pork, venison.

- Seafood: Mackerel, tuna, shrimp, halibut, herring, crab, lobster.

- Dairy products: Yogurt, cheese, milk, cream.

- Fresh fruit: Avocados, cherries, mango, pineapple, oranges, mandarins, bananas, kiwi.

- Fresh vegetables: All green vegetables, spinach, parsnips, mushrooms.

- Nuts: Small amounts of high-fat nuts such as peanuts, almonds, and cashews.

- Whole grains: Bulgur, barley, red rice, corn, oats.

- Legumes: Chickpeas, cannellini beans, fava beans, French green beans, lentils, lima bean, runner bean, sugar snap pea.

2)   Magnesium: This natural sedative helps your body relax as it controls your adrenaline levels. Your hydration levels are improved with a healthy level of magnesium and your muscles find it easier to relax. Here are the foods that will help you boost your levels:

• Fish: Salmon, cod, herring, mackerel.

• Legumes: Small red bean, kidney bean, frijol bola roja, green and yellow peas, alfalfa.

• Dark leafy vegetables: Kale, mustard greens, cabbage, broccoli, arugula, chard, collard greens.

• Bananas

• Low-fat dairy products: Goat cheese, cottage cheese, yogurt.

• Grains

• Dried fruits: Raisins, cranberries, dates, pineapple, apricots.

3)   Calcium: We are all aware of the need for calcium to help strengthen teeth and bones, but did you know it can also help you sleep? Calcium will help your brain process tryptophan to produce melatonin that aids sleep. It also regulates blood pressure and improves muscle contraction and expansion.

These calcium-rich foods will help prevent insomnia:

• Chinese cabbage: Bok choy, Pak Choy.

• Soy products: Tofu, soybean, soymilk.

• Okra

• Cruciferous leafy greens

• Edible green leaves: Dandelion, red clover, watercress, chickweed, plantain.

● Oily fish; Anchovies, herring, tuna, salmon.

4)   B6: Your body needs serotonin. This is a neurotransmitter that promotes sleep and regulates sleep cycles. Vitamin B6 helps the brain to convert a small amount of tryptophan into serotonin. These foods will help you keep you maintain a healthy level of B6 in your diet:

● Organic meat: Steak, beef, venison, chicken, pork, mutton, lamb.

● Seafood: Swordfish, lobster, cod, halibut, mussels, salmon.

● Dried fruits

● Avocados

● Cruciferous leafy greens: Kale, mustard green, cabbage, broccoli.

● Chickpeas

- Garlic

- Tuna

- Spinach

What drinks can help you achieve a better sleep pattern?

Minerals are not only found in food but also in beverages. A nighttime drink can fit perfectly into your bedtime routine and boost your mineral levels. Drinking one of the following drinks before you go to bed will condition your body to prepare for sleep as well as boosting your mineral levels.

- Warm milk: Filled with calcium and tryptophan; this is the perfect way to trigger the body's natural "sleepy" hormone, melatonin.

• Cocoa: If warm milk doesn't float your boat try cocoa. The Mayans were one of the first people to drink cocoa and prepared it with roasted cocoa beans, hot water, and spices.

• Chamomile tea: The lack of caffeine and the gentle flavor means that chamomile is great for relaxing the mind and body. It calms the nerves and settles the stomach making it a perfect way to prepare for bed.

• Passionfruit tea: Another delicate drink that soothes the nerves, passionfruit tea is packed with healthy minerals.

• Valerian tea: Made from essential oils obtained from the roots of the valerian plant this herbal tea promotes healthy sleep and can also decrease stress. This tea is especially effective for women with menstrual problems.

● Tart cherry juice: This is the best source of natural melatonin.

If you want to sweeten any of the above drinks use honey instead of refined sugar and add a healthy dose of natural sweetener.

Food and drinks to avoid

● Alcohol: Many people believe a nightcap will help them sleep, but in reality, it will interfere with your sleep cycles.

● Caffeine: Avoid all caffeine after 2 pm to help you aid sleep. There are some surprising sources of caffeine, here are some products you may not realize contain caffeine: Energy water, pain relievers, regular and diet sodas, chocolate, and decaf coffees. Decaf products are not necessarily caffeine free, check the levels of all these products.

- Fast food: All fast food will take longer to digest than healthy snacks. If food is lying in your stomach it will prevent you from relaxing properly.

- High-fat foods

- Spicy foods

- Refined carbs: Bread, white rice, cakes, cookies, crackers, pie, and candy.

- PASTA

- NICOTINE

If you need a snack before bedtime, there are a couple of great recipes that are healthy and will not interrupt your sleep. Try these healthy evening snacks for a feel-good factor before bedtime.

Conclusion

Thank you again for downloading this book!

I hope this book was able to help you to understand what is Sleep Apnea and how best to tackle it. Sleep Apnea is both a dangerous yet treatable disease. If left untreated, it can cause multiple problems. But a timely observation of Sleep Apnea and the initiation of its treatment is always recommended. You have been provided with crucial and essential information about Sleep Apnea.

The next step is to be vigilant and make sure that you are not suffering from this condition. Sleep Apnea is on the rise. Especially in the US, Sleep Apnea has affected more than 25 million people. And a disease thatș does not differentiate between kids and adults needs to be taken seriously.

Thank you and good luck!